GOLFERS & SKIERS

Mike Dunn

The Passion for Golfing and Skiing

This book is about passion. Specifically, it is about the insatiable passion for the sports of golf and skiing. It is for those who are driven to spend their weekends, vacations and build houses to be near their sports. Innumerable others spend more than a few moments thinking about one or both of these sports each day.

Many of us smile when we relish fond memories of momentary personal grandeur. We reminisce over the good times with family and friends and fixate on how we can improve by tweaking our technique or tactics.

By comparing these sports, you will advance insights on your quest for improvement; gain understanding or acceptance of your compulsion; boost your motivation to get out there more often, or simply sojourn to a happy place.

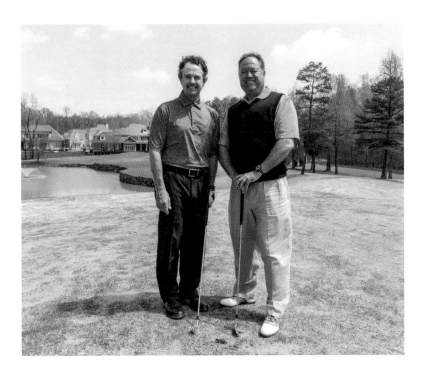

Mike Dunn (right) - author
David Ross (left)– Former PGA Tour Competitor and
Current Golf Director at River Run County Club (home of the Chiquita Classic)

This book is about you rekindling your memories of your friends and family and improving your understanding and skills in golf and skiing. Mike has coached and taught sports for years as an amateur and semi-professional. His favorite phrase is, "Do what I say and not what I do." Sometimes it is self-deprecating, but sometimes not. Over the years, he has amassed a couple of amateur national podiums and many sports trophies, including golfing and skiing. However, like many of you, injuries have throttled his high-end achievement, but not his passion.

He became more and more successful using linkages with demonstrations and word pictures between sports speeding and deepening the athlete's understanding. It was soon apparent that the similarities of golfing and skiing were off the chart. He started documenting the similarities and Golfers and Skiers was born.

Enjoy.

I look forward to golfing and skiing with you soon!

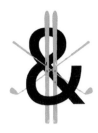

Table of Contents

Preface

The question I am most frequently asked about this book is, "How did I get the idea to write a book on this topic?"

Looking back, the genesis of this concept leveraging the value of comparing skiing and golfing was proven effective years ago when in college. I was then a full time student but worked as a ski instructor in the winter and a tennis instructor in the summer. However, I played golf many weekends and evenings in the spring and summer.

The one thing that set me apart from others in teaching sports, and in my business career, was that I would ask the student or customer many key questions before we got started to maximize the value of our time together. Questions I would ask in skiing lessons were, "What other sports did you do? And what is your level?" I realized if I could articulate and demonstrate the similarities the learning process would be far more effective, yield much faster progress, and the student/customer was much happier after our time together.

If the student was having trouble understanding something even after a skiing demonstration of the drill or turn, I would ask them again which sports they played. Then I would relate the moves back to the sport of skiing. I quickly realized that when someone said they were a golfer, I could come up with a long list of unexpected similarities to explain my points. The golfers that I taught quickly got it and were more confident at the end of their skiing lesson. To a 19 year old kid in college that meant: happier customers = more tips = more money for beer and dates. The good news and bad news is that math seems to still be valid for 19 year olds today.

I would say, "Show me your hip position at the end of your golf swing. OK, that is the hip position for the beginning, middle and end of a correct and smooth ski turn. There, your hips are now fixed. If you do that in skiing, about ninety percent of the time you will no longer have to muscle your turns. You will let your bio mechanics use the ski as a tool. In other words, you will be the puppeteer and your skis will be the puppet. How does that sound?"

Then I would say, "Show me how much your head moves in a skiing turn?" They would say, "It's not supposed to move." I would respond by saying, "correct, and it is the same in a ski turn. If you watch a pro mogul skier ski bumps, you could put an imaginary wire from the top of the run to the bottom going through their forehead and their head will not bobble at all. It will move in a smooth plane all the way down the bump run. The only difference is in skiing you need to keep your chin up to help keep your hips forward."

In a golf stroke, what do your arms do? They would say, "The arms are just along for the ride and to keep the golf club on plane because the lower body is doing all the work." I would say, "The same in a correct ski turn. They are just there to hold on the poles and need to stay in front of you for balance. If your arms are doing more than that, you are going to have problems. In both sports, your arms do virtually nothing."

I would ask, "What are your wrists doing in your golf swing?" They would say, "The looser they are the better and farther you will hit the ball because you generate more club head speed. If your wrists are tight, bad things will happen." I would say, "Again, skiing is the same. The looser your wrists, the better you will ski. It sounds insignificant but it is actually true. The wrists start the timing of a new turn. If your pole plant is smooth and has rhythm, then there is a better chance your turn will as well. In skiing, loose wrists are a significant key to good bio-mechanical timing – just like in a correct golf swing."

I would ask, "Where is your weight in a golf swing?" They would say, "Barely back to neutral then moving forward to the front foot. But, never back." I would say, "Skiing is the same. In the beginning, you may be slightly back to neutral. Then your weight moves forward to the rest of the turn. In golf, you move forward and stop. However, in skiing, you eventually have to move back to reload so you can move forward again. In both sports, it is a fight to stay forward."

I would then ask, "Where is the power generated in a golf turn?" They would say, "From the torque in the lower body and the core. I would say, "In skiing the torque is generated from the lower body and the core."

Then a few perceptive people would ask, "What is the main difference between the moves in the two sports. I would say, "There is really just one major difference between a correct golf stroke and a correct ski turn. In a golf swing, the shoulders pendulum point where the torque releases since the feet are anchored to the ground in a stationary position with golf spikes. In skiing the shoulders and hips are solid and square therefore the torque releases in the legs, feet and skis. That's it."

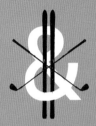

INTRODUCTION

GOLF IS LIKE SKIING. SKIING IS LIKE GOLF.

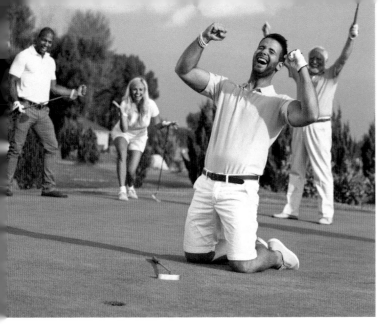
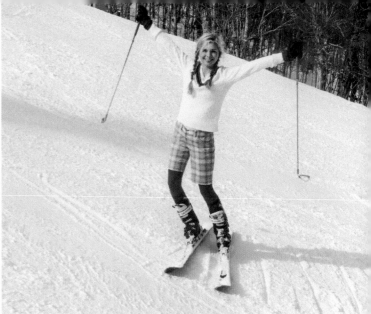

When I was ten years old, I had the good fortune of watching "Slamming" Sam Sneed on the driving range for about thirty minutes. I have never forgotten his slow back-swing and flawless tempo. Without question, the equivalent of "Slammin' Sammy" in the history of the snow ski racing world is Ted "Shred" Ligety. Watching Ted on a giant slalom course gave me a feeling of awe as powerful as watching Sam Sneed practice golf. Ted rode the sharp edges of his skis so cleanly with near zero slipping and such smooth transitions, that it looked as if he were shredding a white piece of paper with his ski edges.

Naturally, I had to learn both sports. I can clearly remember some of my best golf shots from decades ago as if they had happened yesterday. Some were great because of the result or score. Others were great because of the praise I was given for a good shot and still others were great because of the high drama of the situation. Above all, my most memorable golf shots gave me that euphoric feeling of a pure strike of the ball. I also remember making just eight epic turns on skis before a group of high-level skiers in two feet of perfect snow and the sincere compliments following my performance. All were former west coast skiing instructors. One said, "How did you learn to ski like that on the east coast?" I said, "Lots of airline tickets." Both sports are addicting in pursuit of the pure feeling of near perfection. It is an addiction that makes grown men and women spend vast amounts of wealth and precious time on this earth trying to relive, equal, or surpass that feeling.

Both sports offer life lessons that enhance both your personal and professional life if you are willing to open your eyes and mind. One of my favorite aphorisms in my life that has helped my through difficult times is, "Over 51 percent of the putts left short, don't go in." (– Anony-mous). To me this meant to do the extra five percent on an activity to be successful. Late on a Friday afternoon, I would make that extra sales call or ask the extra question to gain further understanding from a friend in need, or a customer. In other words, there is often just a fine line between success and failure.

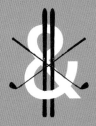

PART I:

THE SPORTS AND THE PEOPLE

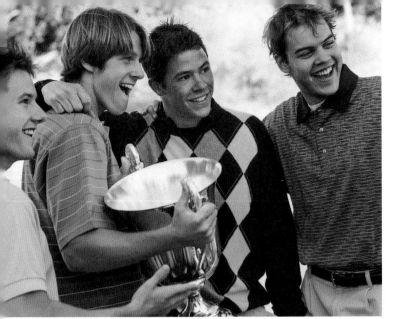 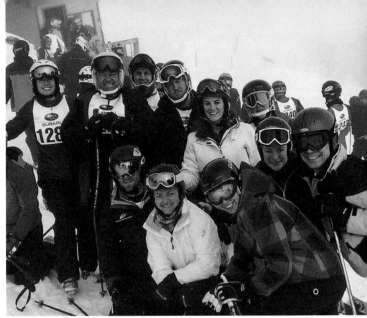

G olf and skiing are social and competitive sports. In both golf and skiing, more time is spent waiting in line than doing the sport. Perfect conditions with no one in front of the golfer or skier are usually found only on TV, or perhaps sometimes on a weekday. The reality is that groups of eager participants must take turns. The finest ski resorts and golf clubs spend millions of dollars to reduce the wait for patrons as much as possible, while also making those unavoidable lift-line and backed-up golf hole delays as pleasant as possible.

But these conditions provide friends and family members with relaxed visiting time. In addition, business associates can find in golf (a warm-weather sport) or skiing (a cold-weather sport) relaxed and informal conditions year-round in which to explore a new idea, pitch a sale, or size up a newly-promoted corporate executive. There is nothing like a blue-sky, snow-packed ski day spent with friends in back-county terrain, or a sweet summer's afternoon on the golf course to push current skill level limits and establish comfortable work and leisure relationships at the same time.

Golf and skiing require skills of opposites

How people ever manage to learn golf is amazing to me. It is a confusing game fraught with counter-intuitive movements. Here is a partial list of the madness:

- To make the ball go high, you need to hit down on it.
- To make the ball stay low, you need to lift up on it as you hit it.
- To make the ball go to the right you need to swing to the left.
- To make the ball go to the left you need swing to the right.
- To make the ball go further, you need to swing smoother.
- To hit the ball out of the sand, you don't hit the ball – you only hit the sand instead.
- The less you move your feet or your head, the better your golf-shot result.

Skiing is also filled with contradictions and counter-intuitive movements that separate poor skiers from high--level amateurs and professionals.

- To turn right, you need to lean to the left or at least be straight from the core up. Your body makes the shape of a "C".
- To turn left, you need to lean to the right or at least be straight from the core up. Your body makes the shape of a "C".
- To turn right, press hard on your left foot while you are still turning right.
- To turn left, press hard on your right foot while you are still turning left.
- When out of control, press hands and body forward, resisting the urge to go backwards.
- When it is extra steep, you need to lean even "further" down the hill.
- To keep your feet warmer in your ski boots, you need to wear thinner socks.
- Stay centered on your skis without leaning back in rough terrain even though it is natural your mind thinks it is safer to lean back.
- On ice, be light on the edges without extra pressure to keep from sliding out.
- While skiing among trees, look at the space between the trees and not at the trees.
- In skiing a wide-open bowl in flat light, ski on the edge to compensate for the contrast.

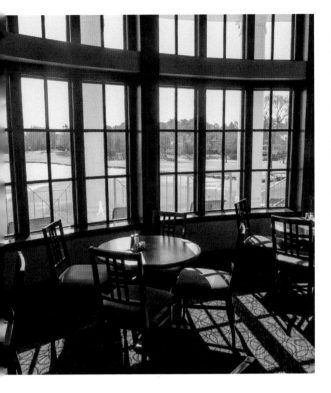 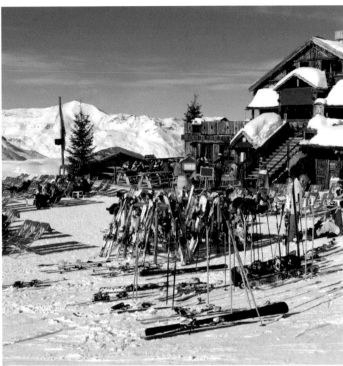

19th Hole and Après Skiing

Both sports wind up at the end of the day at a 19th hole or an après-ski "watering hole". According to Golf info Guide by Thomas Golf, (www.golf-info-guide.com) there are over 15,500 golf clubs in the United States. It would be safe to say that almost every single one has what they would consider to be a 19th hole. Most 19th holes are the bar with the heavy dark wood in a stately room overlooking the 18th green. However, most of the aforementioned bars have a closed-off invitation only back room, for card games and other rumored activities. That, in many instances, that is the real 19th hole.

How do you compete with 11,600 19th holes in the US? By having whole towns mostly dedicated to après skiing. For example, the town of Whistler, BC has 100 bars and restaurants in one square mile area. The town of Aspen has been legendary as an intense party town for the rich and famous. With its close driving distance to Denver and the large army of Summit County ski resort workers, the town of Breckenridge, Colorado is well known as the best party town for the under-forty crowd. The most intense on-slope party I have ever experienced was at the top of the Wengen, Switzerland's world cup course. Beside the train station at the base of the Eiger was a 50 foot tall American teepee. The Swiss totally put the après ski parties in North America to shame.

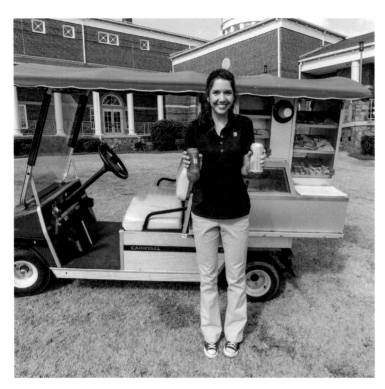 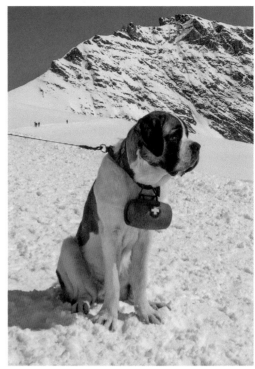

Cocktail concierge to go is unique to both sports

PS: Runner up the 19th hole and Après skiing. The beloved golf cart girls selling beer and snacks while you and your group finish putting will always put a smile on your face. Right after the Masters in Augusta is over, the golfing aficionados know to go to TBonz on Washington Street. It's where all the winning caddies go for an intense reception and party. Skiing has the mythical St. Bernard with the toddy cask around his neck. I have skied in most resorts in the US and many in Europe. I hope to see one in real life with real booze in the cask. Even more legendary than TBonz, is the A-Basin Beach. It is actually just the parking lot at the A-Basin Ski Resort in Summit County, Colorado. Every weekend, hundreds of tailgaters cookout after skiing. Many see the need to have hot-tubs in the back of their pickup trucks. Since hot tubs include bikinis, the math is simple.

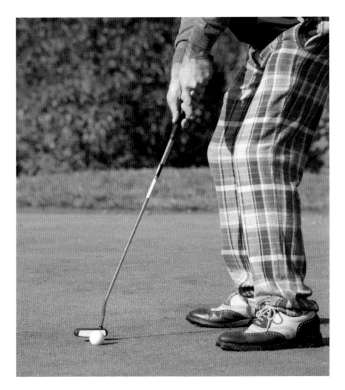 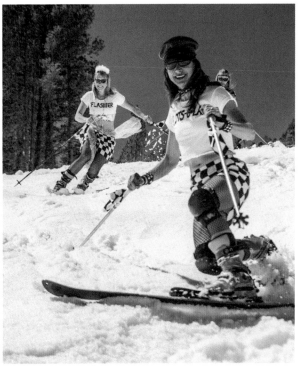

Both sports involve funny-looking clothes and shoes

At least one glove is required; well, that would be just one in golf. The appropriate attire on the slopes and at the green is well-known for being over the top. From the late Payne Stewart's knickers to the bright "snow bunny"(Suzy Chapstick) ski attire of the 1980s to the Fuxi speed suits of today, golfing and skiing are "display" sports; participants not only come to see, but also to be seen making a "fashion statement".

Building and Creating Relationships

A unique aspect of both golf and skiing is that you are sitting beside someone for long lengths of time. Most likely, you are in a golf cart with someone for an hour of a four-hour round of golf. In addition, there are usually two carts with two other people for even more conversation, humorous stories and comradery. If the course is backed up, it will be even longer. Most ski lifts last from five to fifteen minutes holding two to six people and giving you time to bond with your family members, friends or time to make new friends. Being on a ski lift or golf cart is highly conducive to good conversations and not logistically practical for texting, playing video games or making phone calls. Fathers and sons, mothers and daughters, fathers and daughters, husbands and wives, other family members and friends can strengthen and renew relationships when alone together in a fun environment. Golf and skiing can provide those opportunities. That is one of the great things that make our sports different.

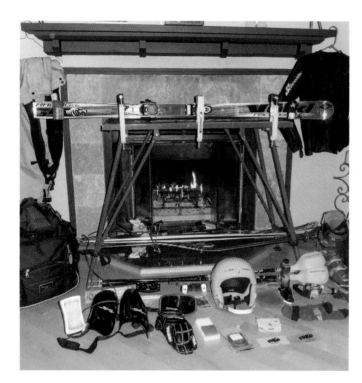
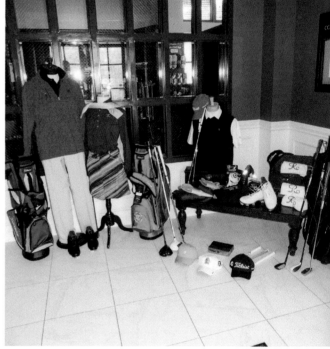

Golf and skiing are equipment-intensive sports

Golfers have golf clubs and are always trying out new gadgets to gain an advantage over their buddies. Similarly, skiers may have many pairs of skis for different situations (GS racing, slalom racing, fast cruising, skiing off-piste, powder, bumps or just social skiing with their intermediate kids, family or friends). They may have several thousand dollars-worth of ski-tuning gear, extra straps for their boots, the latest in body armor, the latest in helmets, flashing jackets, technical jackets, racing suits; the list goes on and on. And so does the money - -easily averaging $3,000 on the conservative side per year is spent on all this gear.

In both sports there is now extensive use of titanium, Kevlar, graphite, GPS for distance to the hole, distance skied or walked and vertical drop skied.

Regulatory bodies throttle equipment innovations in both sports

The USGA (and the R&A) regulates competitive rules and equipment specifications for golf. They regulate which technical advances are legal and which are not.
See FAQ http://www.usga.org/equipment/faq/Equipment-FAQ/#2 to see what is, and what is not, permissible. A stated reason for controlling which equipment and ball advances need to be regulated is the fact that it is not in the best interests of the game of golf to have equipment that can make golf courses too easy. For example, a huge advantage is a pitching wedge with extra grit from sand blasting on the face to enable more spin to stop the ball. The USGA has a rule to set the maximum grit on the face at 180 micro inches of roughness.

FIS is the overseeing body for snow ski racing equipment. FIS's major change for all racers above NASTAR level is that for skis to be FIS compliant, they now cannot be fully-parabolic, or have a radical shape. The primary reason given for this regulation is that skiers have gotten so good at racing on these skies that the G-forces on racers' knees are dangerously high. The new specifications resemble the "old straight skis", which are longer and do not carve as well as parabolic skis. The new FIS legal skis will tend to slide out and chatter more than carve a smooth turn. Hence, if a ski slides out, the G-forces on the racer's knees and legs are reduced. I am proud to say another commonality in both governing bodies is that each has done well to stay away from the negative publicity that has dogged many of the other international and domestic sporting bodies. Generally speaking, the absence of bad news is a trait of good leadership.

When I was 14, my buddy Dallas and I skipped school; which actually rarely happened for either of us. We made our own tickets and snuck into the Kemper Open at Quail Hollow County Club. We walked out of the woods acting like we had just relieved ourselves on the par five 15th fairway. Sam Sneed had just hit his tee shot in some very deep grass beside a lake trying to cut the corner and could not find his ball. I said, "Let's go help him find his ball. " After Dallas jumped into the water looking for the ball, he got out and reached down. As he proudly picked the ball up and held it above his head, he said, "Here it is." Sam's face turned white and the marshal said on the radio, "We need a ruling." I said, "Dallas, we gotta get out of here now." We walked away fast with our homemade tickets spinning in the wind.

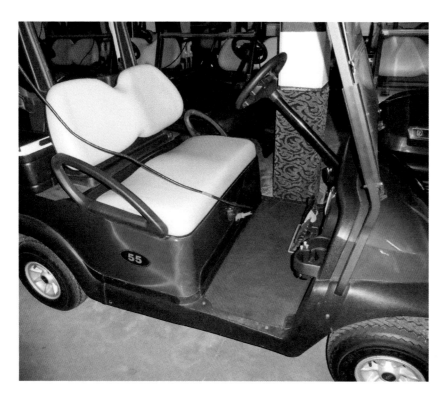
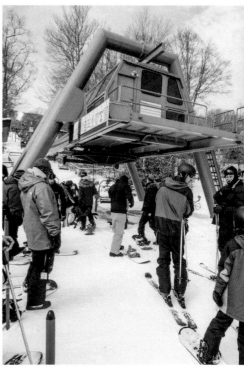

Both sports are electric

Skiing and golf involve taking a motorized transport in the company of another person, which also offers excellent opportunities for great conversations in both the golf cart and the ski lift chair. In the old days, skiers used to hike (walk) and so did golfers. The first ski lift in the world was at Dollar Mountain in Sun Valley, Idaho. They copied cable lifts that transported bananas over the jungle to the transport loading docks for overseas shipments. From there, resorts installed two-person lifts, gondolas, trams, rope tows, platter lifts, detachable quads, detachable six-person lifts and even escalators for the little kids. Golf kept it simple: golfers could drive either a gas or electric cart from green to green; now equipped with a GPS, if desired.

You know you're in trouble when your buddy is driving the golf cart and it's on two wheels. Even worse, you know you're REALLY in trouble when you are looking down at the lake from above the roof. I'm just saying….

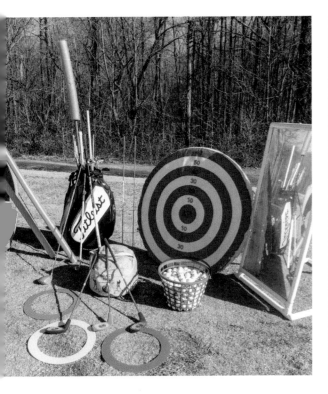 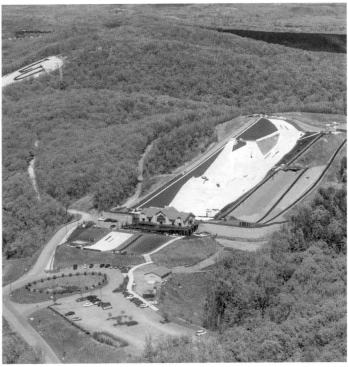

Both invest almost as much in instruction as in instructional gadgets

There are thousands of golf and skiing instructors in the world. Per the "White Book of Ski Areas.com" and "www.Golf-Info-Guide.com" there were '"unofficially" over 18,500 golf clubs and 655 ski resorts in North America alone; nearly all of which have golf teaching pros and ski schools.

Selling golf teaching gadgets is a multi-million dollar industry. You have thousands of practice balls at the driving ranges at most every golf course. The use of practice balls is a significant source of revenue at most public golf courses. In addition, you can buy plastic balls, balance boards, shafts with a hinge, kid's plastic clubs, foam to keep your elbows together, mirrors that do not break, things to keep your head still, giant circular rings to keep your swing on plane, and much more. Then, add the videos for all these gadgets and the other videos from most every big name or famous coach in professional golf and it all adds to big dollars.

Not to be outdone, in skiing we have fake mountains, which are actually real mountains with a wet plastic surface for summer skiing on hot days. Pictured in the upper right is Liberty Mountain Snowflex at Lynchburg University in Lynchburg, Virginia. It is actually realistic and quite fun. It rewards correct fundamental skiing and provides negative reinforcement in the form of rug burns for those who insist on skiing "their way."

My favorite pair of skis met their demise on the backside of a mogul at Lake Louise, AB. The front and top looked perfect. The backside was dry granite. I had no chance.

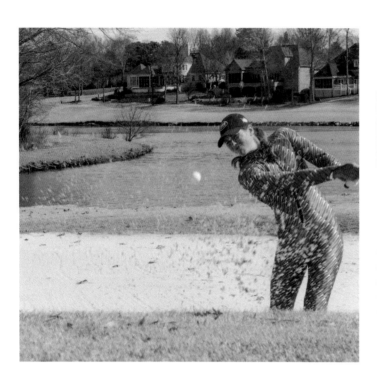 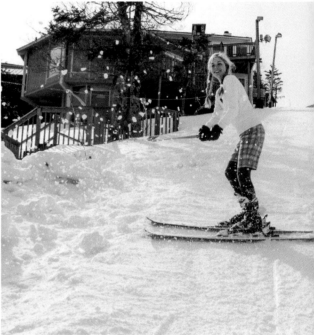

Iconic Balls

Golf balls are the iconic, top of mind, symbol for the sport of golf. The small, uniform, and usually white sphere is recognized in most places on the planet. Most amateur golfers know that golf balls are essentially rented. In other words, you will eventually lose them, only to be found by another golfer, enterprising kids, or a person who probes the many lakes and ponds on courses throughout the land. The golf ball divers use diving gear to find the mother-load of golf balls to re-sell to bargain-hungry high handicap golfers. As the unofficial story goes from Florida, locals (it appears the real story with the names is under non-disclosure per the locals), a golf ball diver took a week off to go dive on a boat with some treasure hunter for no pay, off the coast of Key West in July of 1985. On our golf ball diver's first dive, he found the largest treasure find since King Tut's tomb. The Captain was Mel Fisher's son, Kane, and the wreck was the Spanish ship Atocha. The "unnamed" contingency crew got their split. It was worth

400 million dollars. After years of litigation, it "appears" the official story has changed. So pick the version of the story you want to believe.

Like golf, balls are also the iconic reference in skiing – in this case, snow balls. All kids on earth in areas that get snow make snowballs. All college freshmen from the state of Florida who go to northern schools make snowballs. The number of snowballs made by each person in their life can be an inverse relationship to that person's maturity level. Please list the names of the fine people who come to mind in that category in the right hand margin on this page.

The other white gold is snow, which is turned into hundreds of thousands of lift tickets each year. Like snorkelers searching for golf balls, skiers in very deep white gold (dry snow) nearly need snorkels to breathe in the powder flowing over the skier's head

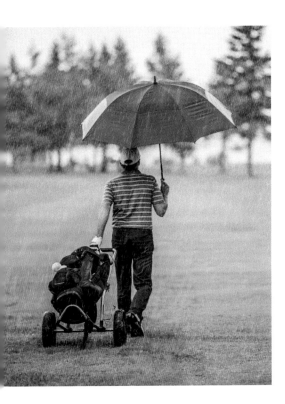 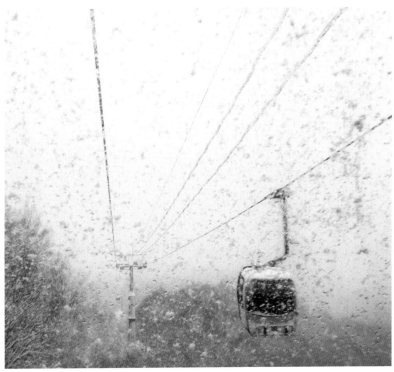

Both sports take up a whole day out in the weather

Both golfing and skiing are completely weather-dependent activities with varying conditions; sometimes on a hole-by-hole or run-by-run basis. At Amen Corner at Augusta National during The Masters, a wind can strike true fear in the hearts of the world's best golfers. Similarly, a small patch of soft snow can cause terror in the hearts of downhill skiers, as one ski sticks and the other may ride free. Rain, fog, wind, extreme cold, heat and even sun and shade can alter tactics, strategies, or approaches to every run or round. Weather is more than just an incidental factor; it is really part of the sport. In golf, changing wind, dampness, dryness, rain and wind-gusts determine continuous changes in tactics and strategy. In skiing and ski racing, a changing wind, snow water content, direction of the sun, shade, rain, snow, sleet, fog, light conditions and ruts determine tactics and strategy for every run or few turns.

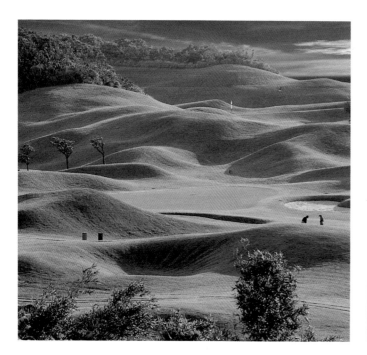 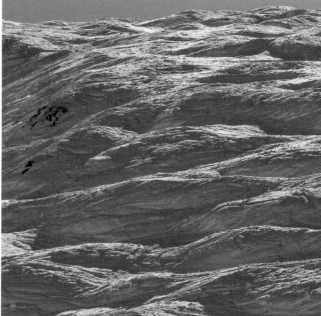

The ups and downs make it fun

Both golf and skiing are highly concerned about the terrain. The changing terrain determines tactics and strategy every bit as much as changes in weather. For golf, the slope of the green or fairway has a dramatic influence on club and shot selection. In skiing, the steepness of the slope or slope features such as moguls completely determine the options of turns from which the skier can choose for safety or effectiveness.

Downhill or side hill lies, in golf with the ball above or below your feet are far more difficult than a perfectly flat lie. However, if it were too easy, it would not be fun. That is easy to say if you don't have a bet with your buddies on the hole.

Skiing moguls (called "bumps" by expert skiers) is challenging, but very fun. With skiing bumps, there are eight things you need to do, and you'd better do at least six of them correctly, or you are in for a long run; your confidence is shot and your day has ended. It takes most people about four days in the bumps each season before they start to regain their timing. But once you've spent your time at it, your skiing confidence doubles and you have a rekindled "bump addiction". You start to view groomed runs as just a way to get you to harder terrain that is more fun. As always, professional ski lessons for moguls or steeps cuts your learning time and pain endured by a significant amount.

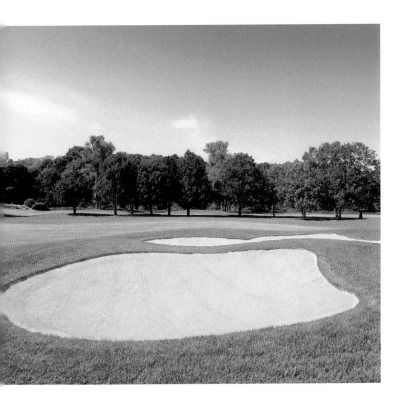 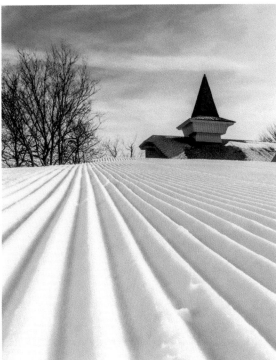

Both industries strive for a smooth playing surface

At nearly every golf course, the grounds-keeping crew is kept busy with a fleet of large and expensive lawn mowers to keep the course manicured and smooth. All skiing resorts have $250,000 snow-cats that smooth out the snow into a velvety corduroy texture for maximum grip, smoothness and bliss. Most resorts have their most trusted employees drive the snow-cats all night to groom slopes into perfection for their paying patrons to enjoy each day. Unless you own one of the other 18,449 golf clubs, I'm sure you would agree that one of the best golf course in the world is Augusta National in Augusta, Georgia - the location of "The Masters". Many of you have heard that photos and TV pictures simply cannot convey the manicured perfection of this golf course during tournament week. It's the only place I've ever seen where a bunch of men in green blazers and starched shirts walk the course at 7:00am (I assume that they were members and not workers) and use 15 foot long flexible rods to knock the dew off the fairways.

I was one of fifty or so lucky people to watch Phil Mickelson make two attempts to get a ball out of a sand trap the day he won the Masters for the first time.

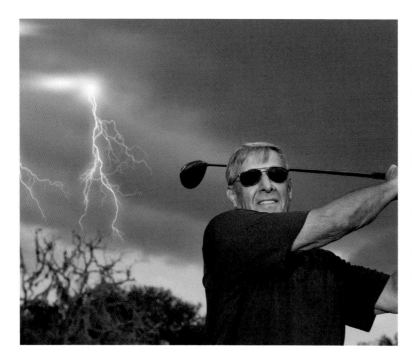 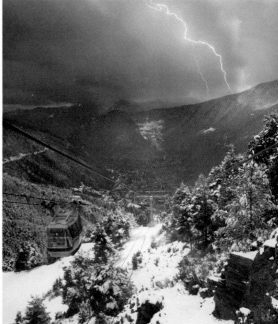

Lightning is a major issue in both sports

Golf is the second-most dangerous sport for lightning casualties; certainly skiers face similar concerns, as some very intense snowstorms produce lightning. The dangers of lightning for golfers are obvious: the players are outside with metal shafts in their hands, either in exposed areas or under trees. Ski conditions for a lightning strike are not as obvious, but could be even more dangerous. Skiers are stuck in metal chairs on a metal cable held up by 40' tall metal poles, while holding metals poles in their hands for five to fifteen minutes. Then they are usually dumped out at the top of a mountain. Thunder snow is rare; however, it does happen in especially intense winter storm conditions. If you hear thunder during a snow storm (or a sleet storm), keep in mind that heavy snow suppresses sound. Therefore, there is a good chance that the lighting is closer than you would expect with the same relative sound of a normal thunderstorm while raining. Statistically, the most dangerous activity during a thunderstorm is water sports (boating, fishing, and swimming). Golf is statistically the second most dangerous activity in a thunderstorm. The United States has the most lighting strikes per year than any other country in the world. The state with the most annual lighting strikes and deaths from lighting strikes is Florida, by a large margin.

My luckiest shot was on a cold winter day when I was in middle school. My sliced five iron approach shot slid across a fully-iced over pond. The ball stopped on five foot wide circle of land in the middle of the pond with a fifty foot long and thirty inches wide walkway to it. I chipped onto the green for a par.

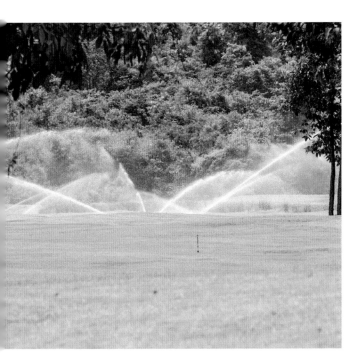
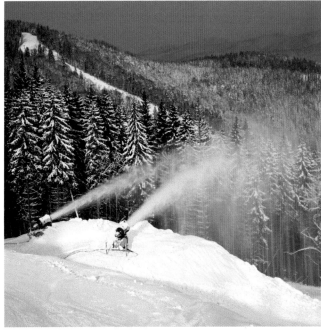

Both sports are water-intensive

It takes lots of water, water pipes, water compressors and sprayers to keep the golf course watered and grass growing. A golf course without enough water means the golfer will be hitting off "hard pan", which is bad for business. Water is even more important in skiing, since snow is frozen water. Moreover, nearly all ski resorts have water reserves, pipes, compressors and sprayers to make snow when Mother Nature supplies the cold air but not enough snow. Hitting golf balls on hard dry ground is not much fun and can harm your equipment. Skiing over a hidden piece of hard dry ground is even worse.

As luck would have it, when you are doing well in your round the fairway or green sprinklers will turn on via the timer. Even worse, if you can imagine, the lift seems to only stop when you are beside a snow gun pasting you with frozen water and chemicals. Unless you are sure you have just completely extinguished your bad luck, you may want consider not gambling or investing in the lottery on days when the aforementioned happens.

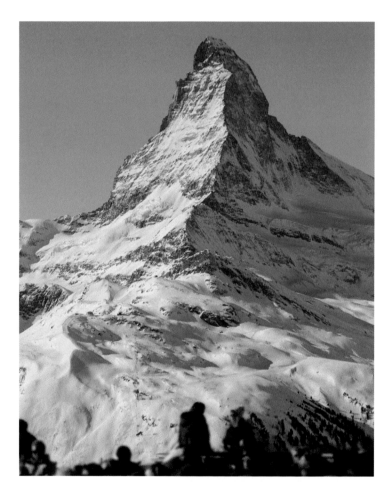

The Matterhorn, Switzerland
(Augusta National not pictured for trademark reasons)

Hallowed Places

By many, Augusta National is considered to be the Mecca or Jerusalem for those who love the game of golf. The first impression most everyone has when they first the Masters is, "I'm in awe that this place is so perfect." The other statement most all newcomers say is, "TV just cannot show the intense beauty of the course." It is hard to find a blade of grass that is out of place or a piece of debris lying around. The Masters is the perfect place to be for both golfers and non-golfers who are OCD. The history and golfing horrors at Amen Corner are something most golf-lovers know well. It is called Amen Corner because it is the end of a string of extremely hard golf holes. Competitors are relieved to get to the last few holes because they are less stressful. The crowds of thousands are reverent when the times warrant and then become silent for the next player's shot. The old school tradition is driven home when you buy a BBQ sandwich for $1.25 and a pimento cheese sandwich for $0.75. If you have not been there, this seems trivial but it is not. It serves as just two examples of the attention to detail that is a part of the mystique and aura of The Masters.

Skiing world history is not as clearly defined as in golf. I think it is because skiing has so many sub-sports, so there is no single best place. You have ski areas that have famous downhill race courses, recreational skiing, major resorts, mom and areas, pop hills, cross country skiing trails, back country skiing s, ski areas that specialize in terrain parks, resorts that cater to families, resorts that cater to luxury experience, and resorts that target the ski/party crowd. This is all great, but undefined. At the risk of causing major controversy, here is my list of the best in golf and skiing:

Most Iconic golf course:
>Augusta National in Augusta, Georgia

Golf course on most golfers' bucket list:
>The Old Course at St. Andrews in Scotland

Course revered to provide the biggest golf challenge:
>Teeth of the Dog in Dominican Republic

Most Iconic Mountain to skiing:
>The Matterhorn

Most iconic lift:
>KT-22 at Squaw Valley

Most scenic view in skiing:
>From the rotating restaurant in the James Bond Movie, *Her Majesty's Secret Service*, Schilthorn – Piz Gloria, in Mürren, Switzerland

Best Party Resort:

Whistler, BC (Honorable mention: Breckenridge, CO)

Best Snow on Earth:

Utah TM. Hard to argue with their trademark and license plates.

Most Hell-Skiing terrain:

Alaska

Longest World Cup Downhill Course:

Lauberhorn in Wengen, Switzerland

Biggest Skiable Mountain:

Mauna Kea, Hawai'i. It is bigger than Mt. Everest from the sea floor and has "hike to" skiing in the winter. Trick question to try on your buddies at the bar.

First Ski Lift:

Sun Valley, Idaho

Place where snowmaking was invented:

Connecticut

Biggest manmade ski hill:

Buck Hill, Minnesota. It's a city dump/trash hill that produced Olympic champions like Lindsey Vonn.

Best one dollar hot dog in the universe:

Mallard Head Golf Club

Most famous indoor skiing hill:

Ski Dubai in Dubai, United Arab Emirates

Every golfer has heard this their whole golfing career. Words or pictures cannot fully convey the magnificence of the Masters at Augusta National. I recommend you add attending a practice round at the Masters to your bucket list. The star is the course and the players are secondary there. David Ross won a professional golf tournament at the Teeth of the Dog course in the 1970s.

Defining Movies

Most sports have defining movies using their sport as a back drop. Golf and skiing are not different. Interestingly, in both sports only humorous movies are top of mind. I will take that as a positive.

Golf has the clear favorite movie, Caddy Shack (1980). I would be confident in saying there is a Caddy Shack quote uttered on every one of the 11,600 golf courses in North America every single day of the year they are open. Honorable mention would be Tin Cup (1996).

Skiing also has a clear winner among movies. From the shores of Lake Tahoe is, Hot Dog –The Movie (1984). Like Caddy Shack, it is full of one- liners with a light-hearted plot and sub-plot. The difference between Caddy Shack and Hot Dog – The Movie is that you cannot let little kids watch Hot Dog – The Movie. Honorable mentions for skiing are. Hot Tub Time Machine (2010) or any of the James Bond movies.

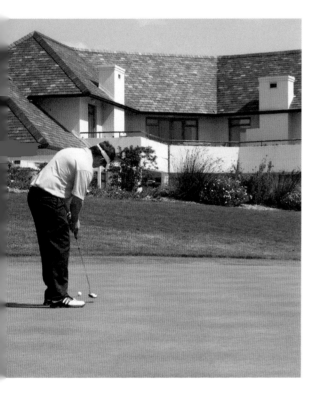 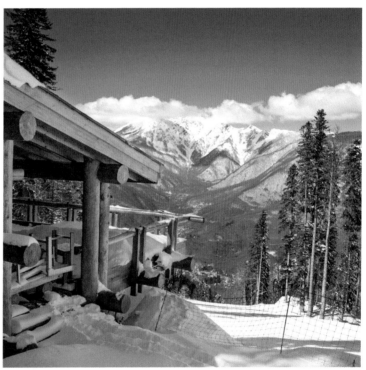

Golfing, Skiing, Lifestyle and Real Estate

Multi-million dollar ski chalets and multi-million dollar mansions on golf courses are the result of passionate and successful like-minded individuals. The luckiest and most focused of all have both. Smart people should always take an assessment of what makes them and their family happy, and then take action. Golf homes, ski chalets, mountain estates and beach homes are the majority of resort property in the world. Passion, family fun and entertaining friends are the drivers in these markets.

Number of Skiing Resorts vs. Golf Courses

Millions of people ski. Many millions of people play golf. Here is a list of golf courses and ski resorts. In addition to places to have fun, these numbers represent multi-billion dollar industries and trillions of dollars in personal wealth.

GOLF COURSES AS OF 2012

Total public golf courses in the U.S. **11,581**

Total municipal owned golf courses **2,449**

Total private golf courses in the U.S. **1,470**

Total golf courses in the U.S. **15,550**

Total number of golfers (2011) in U.S. .... **25.7 million**

Highest number of golfers in U.S. (2003) .... **30.6 million**

Golfers who play 8 – 24 rounds per year .... **14.4 million**

Increase in golf courses since 1990 .... **24%**

Increase in golfers since 1990 .... **17%**

Worldwide golf courses are estimated to be over **30,000**

SKI RESORTS

Europe	1692	**51%**
North America	657	**22%**
Japan	650+	**21%**
Asia (without Japan)	78	**3%**
Australia & New Zealand	55	**2%**
South America	38	**1%**
Africa	7	**<1%**

The "Holy Cow" lift at Telluride lets you ski down a seven-mile-long green run lined with ten- and twenty-million dollar second homes. Most cities and towns have one or two premier county clubs with similar homes. The three most common comments that the masses say about these homes are: 1. "Holy cow". 2. "Where did they get their money". 3. (My personal favorite). "Please adopt me."

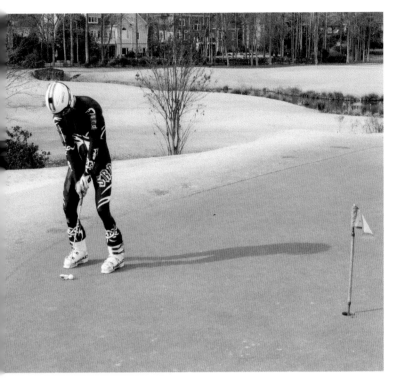
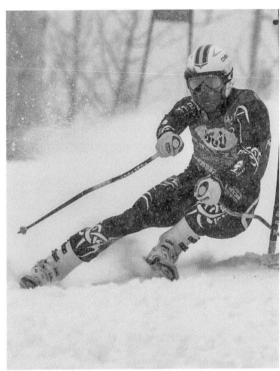

Precision of execution is vital

Golf and skiing are all about precision. In many cases, the margin of error is less than an inch in both sports. In golf it has been said for years that, "You drive for show and putt for dough." Whether you hit a drive 290 yards or 325, it does not matter nearly as much as missing a five-foot putt by one inch or making it. Having more one putt greens, verses three putts, has a dramatic effect on your score and handicap. Skiing is the same. The best case is when you ski exactly the line you want, within inches, at twenty to ninety mph. It is the same in skiing bumps. You want to hit the precise spot to make a turn within a few points. If you are skiing through trees, you had better be precise if you want to live to ski another day. Any mistake or missed turn could result in a sled ride, or the end of the rest of your skiing season and the loss of the spring and summer golfing season.

> *Also at the Kemper Open at Quail Hollow County Club, on the Pro Am day, about seven or eight young boys ran up to Lee Travino on the 2nd tee while he was waiting to hit his tee shot. He said, "Shouldn't you boys be in school?" One kid said, "We came here to see you, Mr. Travino." Lee said, "Why do you want to see me? I'm just a big dummy with a lot of money."*
> *I've loved golf ever since.*

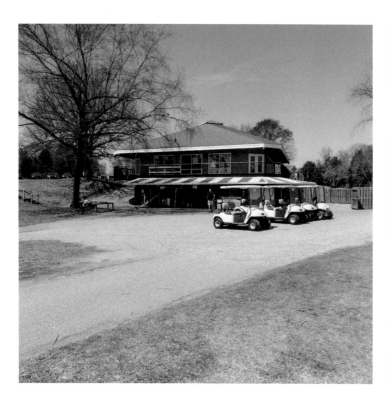

Public Golf Courses and Local Ski Hills

It can be debated that more total fun per day happens on the local public golf courses than at the exclusive private club courses on a day-to-day basis. It also can be argued that there are more golf balls and golf clubs in the water at the local municipal courses. There are just more people who play on the public courses than at the expensive clubs. Since both kinds of courses are fun, it follows that there is more fun realized at the public courses. That being said, most everyone wants to play on a pristine course with little to no backup at the tee box more often found at a county club.

Skiing is similar. Out of only a handful of private ski resorts, almost all ski areas are public. However, even more than golf, all ski areas offer season passes, which is more or less a year's membership. Unless you live near one of the 60 North American mega-resorts, you most likely frequent your local hill and go to a mega-resort two or three times a season. Like golfers who want to play the country club, or the county club that supports a big name PGA tournament, skiers dream about having a powder day at their favorite mega-resort. Fun is had by all.

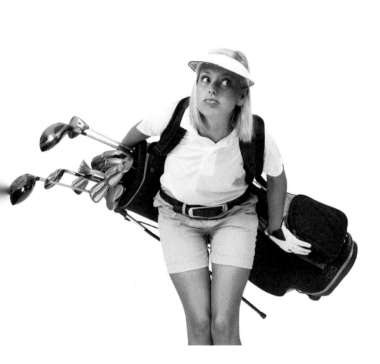
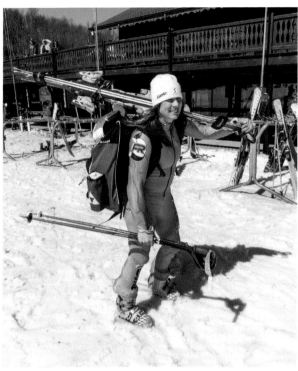

Gear to Carry

Some of the best words that can ever be uttered to a Dad is, "I want to carry my own golf bag or skis." Both sports are very gear- intensive. Golf bags can be huge and ski gear for three can fill up an SUV as well as a golf foursome.

> *On our ski trip to Switzerland, my wife, my ski and golfing buddy and his wife set the record for something. Per the Grindelwald hotel owner, he said we set the record for the most luggage for four people since his family owned the hotel.*

As mentioned before, both sports are gear-intensive. In golf, things are fairly straight forward. You have a big bag with all your stuff in it. You either carry it or roll it. However, you most likely put it on the back of the cart and drive it around. Better yet, you have someone else drive you around in the cart. Also, in golf you usually have a valet get your clubs from you and put them on the cart for you for a small tip. Most all three modes of moving your stuff are appropriate. If you carry your bag often, most likely you will have a smaller and lighter bag as you walk.

Unless you are at Deer Valley, it does not work this way in skiing. You have to carry your heavy skis and sometimes a full boot bag as well a long way to your locker to change. Then, you carry your skis and poles while walking in your boots to the lift. Once you get on the electric powered lift, only then do the similarities to golf return.

Have your friends stop freaking advanced skiers out with this faux pas.

Usually there are few issues involved with carrying golf equipment. Skiing is a whole different matter from an etiquette point of view. If you are in a ski town and watching the local ski channel, you will occasionally see a bit about ski-carrying etiquette. This may not seem like a big deal, but to true skiers it is finger nails on a black board. The TV shows in Aspen will say, "Don't carry your skies like THOSE people in Vail". Conversely, the snow folk in Telluride will say, "We in Telluride never carry our skis like THOSE people in Aspen." What they are saying is, carry your skies in one of two ways. The most approved way, if you are away from crowds, is to put your skis over your shoulders with the tips forward AND with the toe piece of the binding behind your shoulder (pictured above). If you are in a crowd, carry your skis with everyone else in a 100 percent vertical position by holding the toe piece of your binding with your hand. Hint: one way will slip and the other will be secure so you have a 50/50 chance that you will guess right when you pick up your skis this way.

During my twenty-four year career in commercial sales, I have had the good fortune to play many charity golf events a year. I made sure my management and the public relations department knew that I had a list of CIOs and decision-makers agreeable to being called in at the last minute to fill in for other customer cancellations. If my customer played, that meant I was expected to join him or her. There were always last minute cancellations. There is no question that golf builds relationships. I kept most of my largest customers for over twenty years.

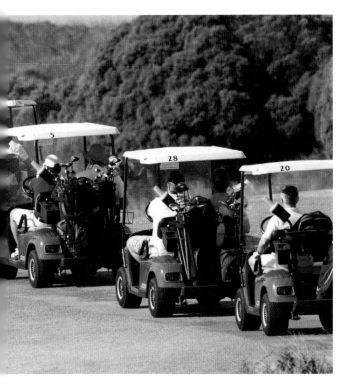
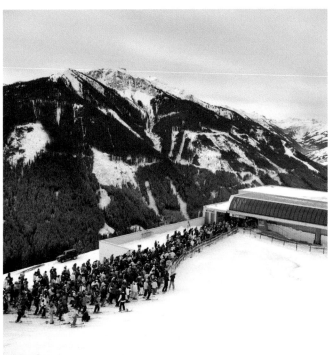

The Waiting

Unless you are a private club member and play on a weekday, you will be resigned to waiting. The better the weather the longer the wait, is the rule of thumb. On a golf course, it takes just one slow player or group of players to delay everyone's day, thus decreasing the fun by some percentage. Golf marshals can have varying degrees of influence to get people to play faster. If you are lucky, the slow players will let you play through, which will ease your frustration somewhat, but then they will still have to deal with the foursome behind you. A busy day with slow players can add thirty minutes to two hours to your round. But a day on the golf course beats working.

Skiing has the dreaded long lift line. During the season, Saturdays between 11am and 2pm are usually the busiest times of the week at most every ski area on the planet. Lines from one to fifty minutes can happen. Once you know a ski area, you can predict where not to be during the day to avoid the lift lines and find the best snow based on conditions like sun, melting, wind and terrain.

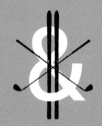

PART II:

GALLERY

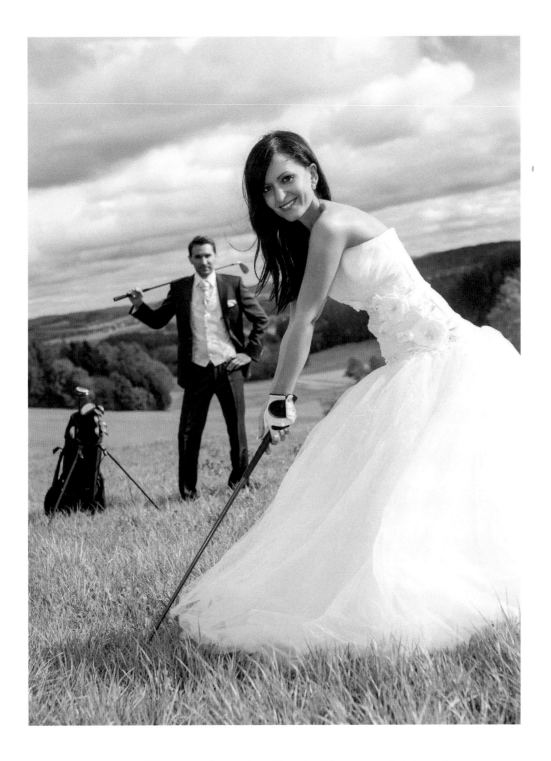

No worries. This was not her real wedding day. The guy was just dreaming...

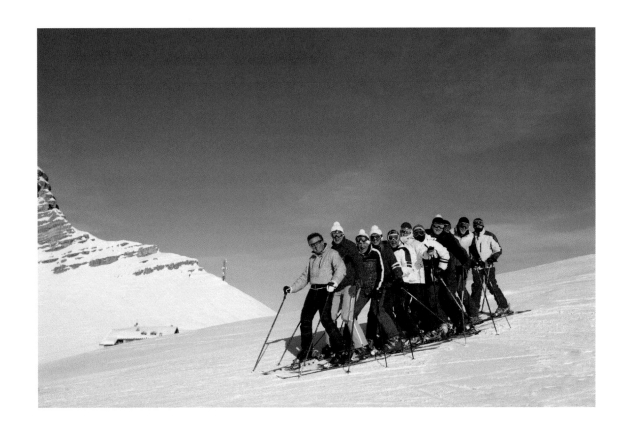

Canadian fun. It is amazing what people do when leaving the on-mountain bar with a camera.

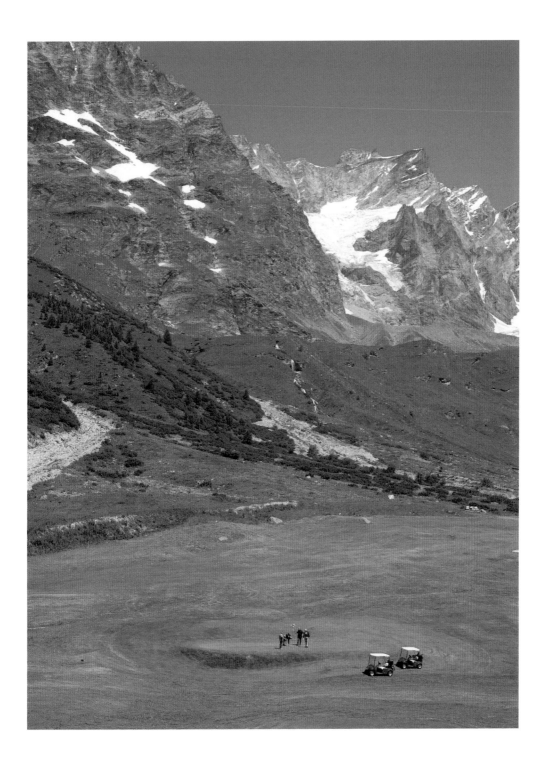

The reason some mountain courses are so hard to play is because the scenery is so stunning you can't keep your head down.

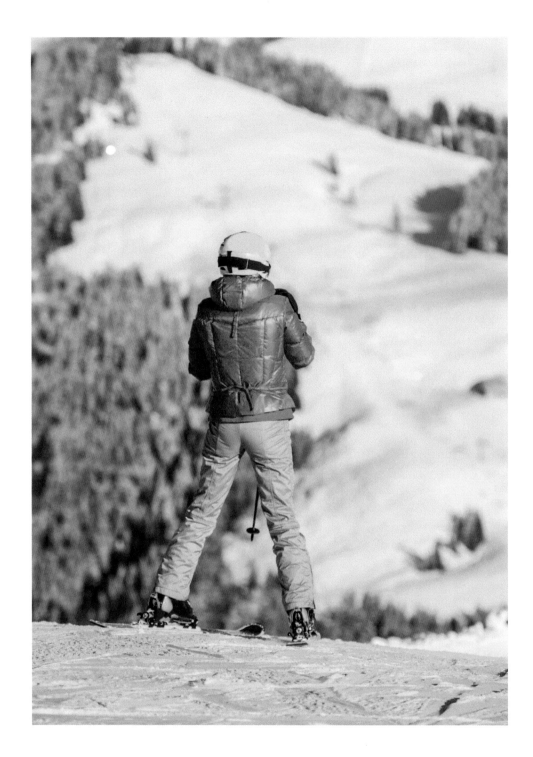

Making a plan before you start a steep run is always a good idea.

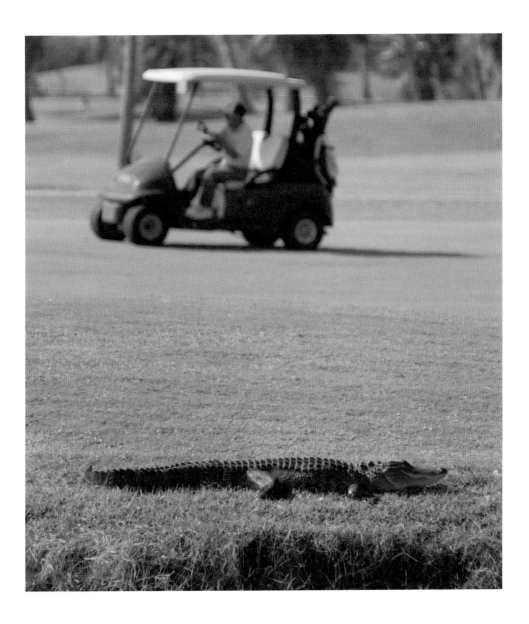

What is your favorite gator, moose, bear or other wildlife golf story? Mine was in Barbados. We were about to tee off when the large branches in a fully-grown tree started to shake violently on a day with only a light sea breeze. Then, three gigantic looking spider monkeys (or gibbons?) walked from the tree crossing the fairway about two hundred yards from the tee box. It could be an exaggeration due to our excitement, but they looked four feet tall. They appeared taller but thinner than chimpanzees. They seemed to keep moving away so we continued our round. I know what you're thinking, but there was no Barbados rum involved since I was golfing with my Dad.

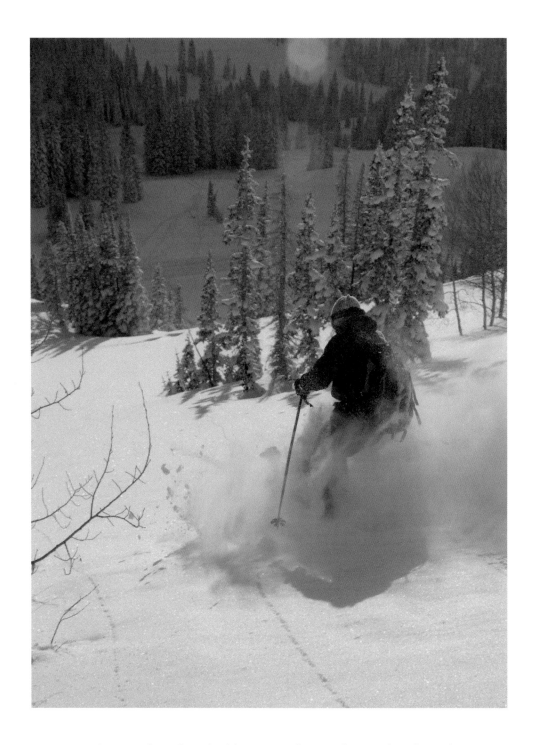

Powder Day Rule #1: If your buddy is running late, you leave without him or her.
Powder Day Rule #2: Every man (or woman) for themselves – see Rule #1

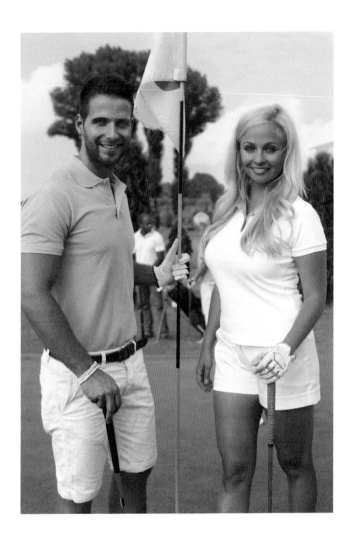

Golfing and skiing are great activities to share with your spouse or significant other. If one of you is a beginner, never, ever teach or be taught by your spouse. Why? If you are the beginner, your husband/boy friend WILL leave you at the top of the mountain or steep slope as a joke. Per Jim Cottrell, author of several books on skiing, this is the main reason people quit the sport of skiing. If you are the affable teacher, nothing you do will be right; it will all be your fault and your day will end in an argument. The solution is easy, sure and clear. The first three times the beginner golfer or skier goes with you, have them take a lesson from a professional golfing or skiing instructor. The instructor can tell your spouse the exact same words, but they will be right and you will be wrong. It will save your day, your relationship and your vacation.

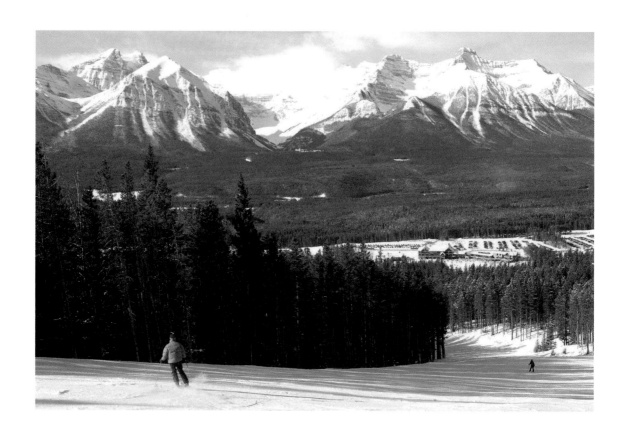

Many say the most scenic ski resort in North America is Lake Louise, AB. I emphatically agree. The last time I was in Banff/Lake Louise, each morning there were fresh elk and wolf prints in the snow around our chalet. In my humble opinion, only Murren, Switzerland has more breathtaking scenery than Lake Louise/ Banff, AB.

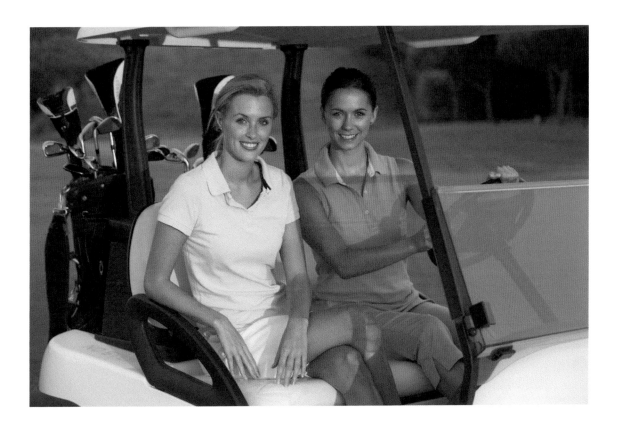

Golf has many wonderful aspects. Not the least of which is the social aspect.

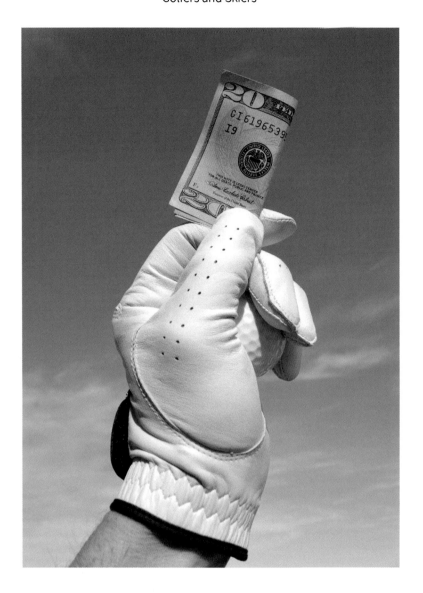

An older friend of mine was transferred by his company from a large city to a small town. Naturally, he bought a house on the local golf course. One weekday morning he was asked to fill in for one of the players in a standing foursome of local business owners. They were playing for a dollar a hole and my friend won five dollars from this one fellow. They all had a beer at the 19th hole and settled up on the bets. Unknown to my friend, his business was a major supplier to a retail chain that had just filed bankruptcy and his company was about to do the same. Apparently, the guy snapped sometime between after the golf round and the next morning. He took one of his cars, drove the next largest town and robbed a bank. The ink exploded in the car, no one was hurt and he was immediately caught. So, I said to my friend in a loud voice, "it's your fault, you took his last $5.00!" Tears of laughter followed. His customary birthday and Christmas present from me is a funny card with a five dollar bill.

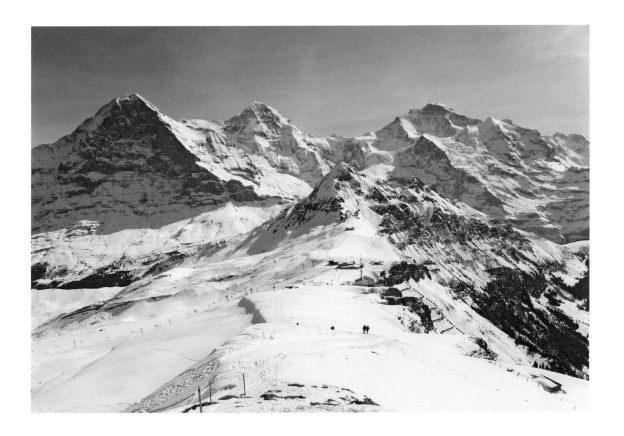

Intimidation. The longest downhill course on the World Cupp circuit each year is the Laubenhorn in Wengen, Switzerland. It is a thigh-burning, thirty- to forty-five seconds longer than any other downhill. It has the longest jump on the circuit, as well as the only downhill race where the racers approach 100 mph. After skiing the course with some locals, for me, the most terrifying part is near the top. As the racers leave the start and descend down the steep bowl, they approach the famous Hundschopf (dog's ears) jump at near 90 mph. If that is not terrifying enough, the racers must go between two massive granite outcroppings; each the size of a two-story house. The problem is that these two monoliths are just twenty feet apart. At 90 mph, many things can go wrong, especially on skis. The racers are keenly aware that if they were to catch an edge two hundred years or meters before the Hundscopf, many bad things could happen.

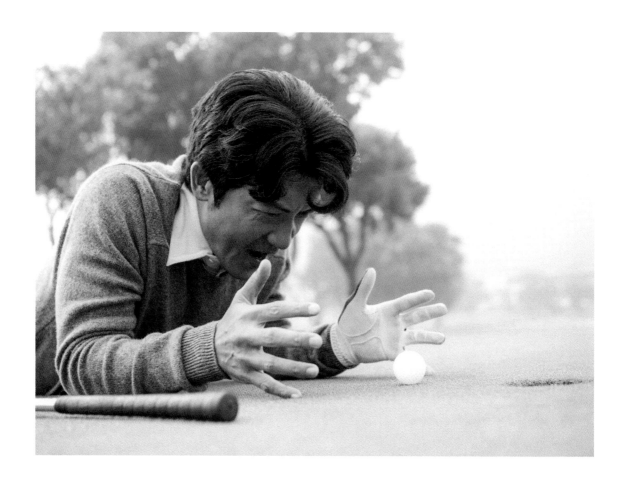

How many golf clubs have you seen heaved into the woods or a lake? My childhood and lifelong buddy has "helicoptered" golf clubs into the woods during meltdowns. He has "helicoptered" tennis racquets over the fence after missed shots. He is legendary. Best of all, he once hit me with a very accurate "helicoptered" ski pole from twenty five yards in Deer Valley while laying on the ground while mostly buried in fresh powder. For the record, I completely deserved being hit with the pole. When he nailed me, the other three of us laughed even harder, if that was possible, at his expense.

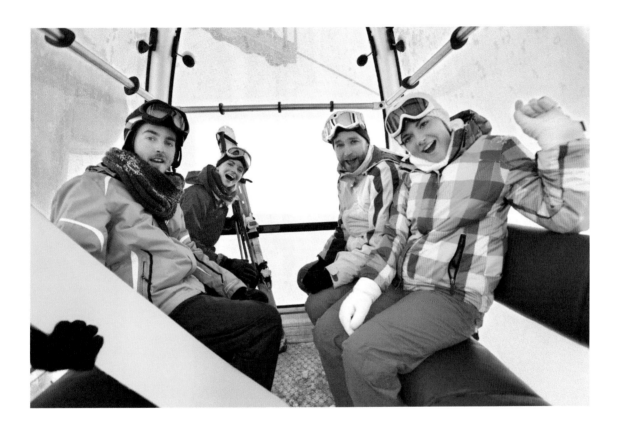

Skiers and boarders enjoying a warm and long gondola ride during a snow storm.

In college, I took skiing as one of my physical education requirements. The surreal part was that I had to fill out the documentation for my official grade, since I was also the skiing instructor for my class. It was only pass/fail so no "A" for me, just a "P".

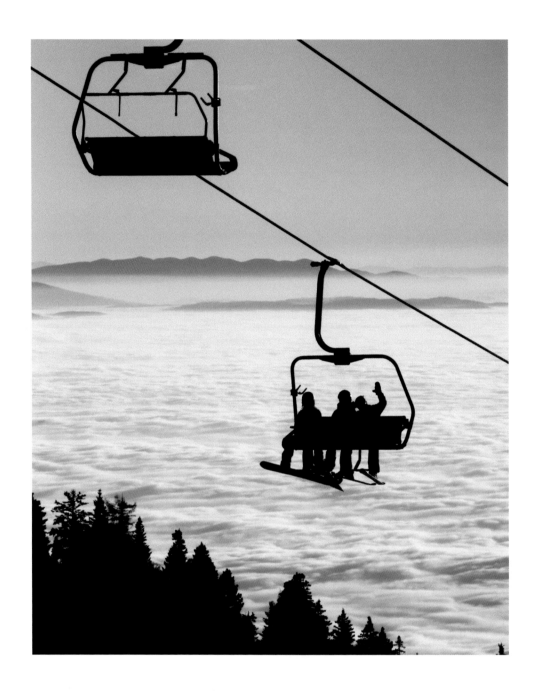

I have never had to be evacuated from a broken ski lift so far in my years of skiing. However, I have been a few chairs from getting on one, or had just gotten off a broken chair three times. Once, I just had to step off at the top. An evacuation involves the ski patrol lowering skiers down to the ground from the chairs on the cable by rope system.
Statistically, I am overdue.

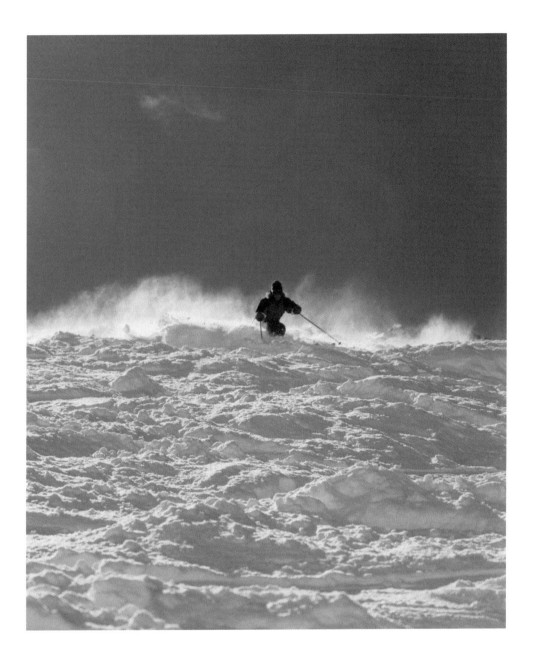

Learn to love chopped powder. How? 1. Keep both shins forward all the time. 2. Pretend you are skiing in a cement culvert that is 8" shorter than your height. Moreover, your head cannot go above that imagery culvert top. When you hit unseen bumps you just suck up them up with your abs, moving your hips and legs forward. 3. Press hard on your outside ski EXTRA early in your turn. Start pressing at the 7 o'clock position. The 9 o'clock at the fall line is far too late. Then, enjoy!

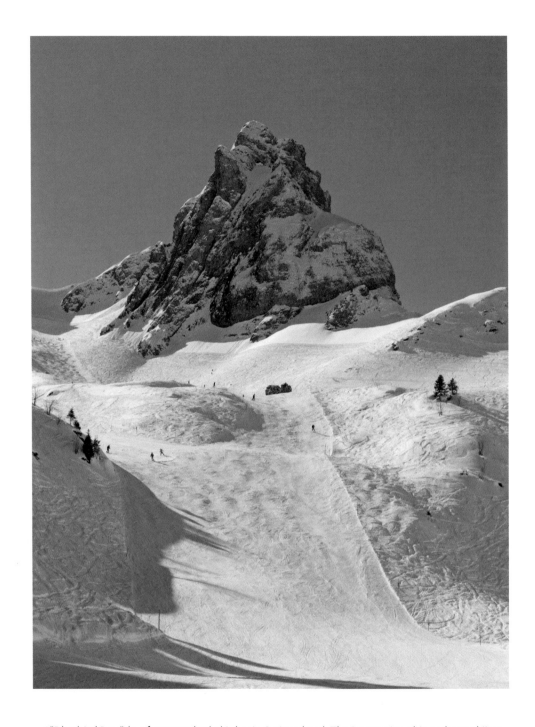

A "Bluebird Day" (perfect weather) ski day in Switzerland. The interesting thing about skiing in Europe is that you can pass several cow barns and barns converted into bars on one five-mile long ski run. Do you know how to tell the difference? The smell.

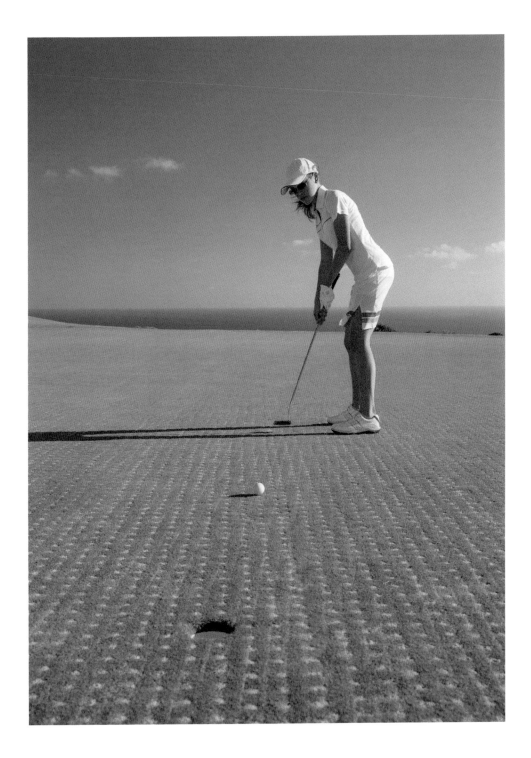

If all aerated greens had this view, no one would ever complain again.

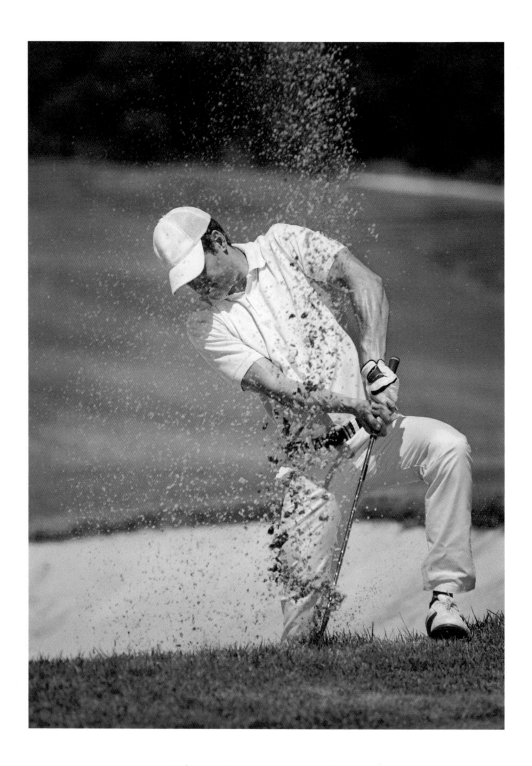

Golf is easy if you never make mistakes.

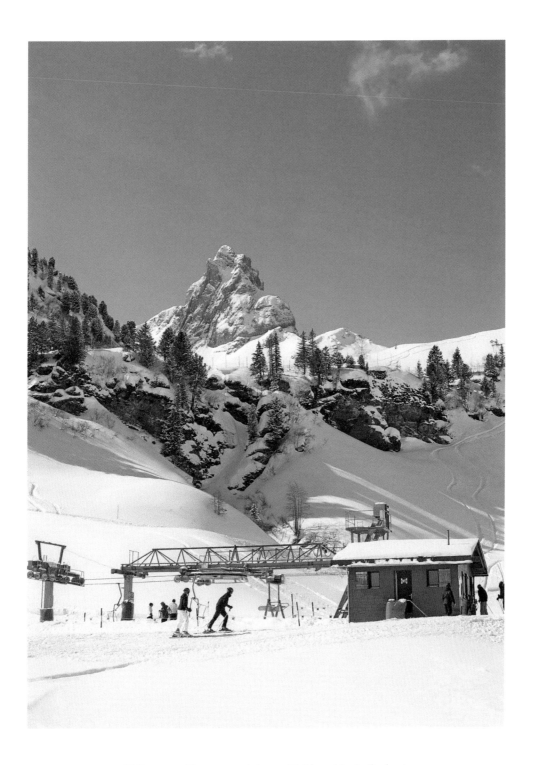

Skiing or golfing on weekdays with blue skies is the best.

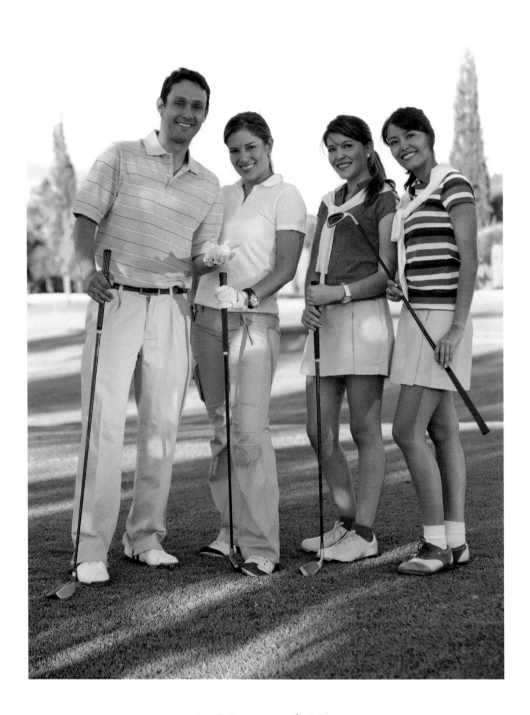

Family Fun on a perfect day.

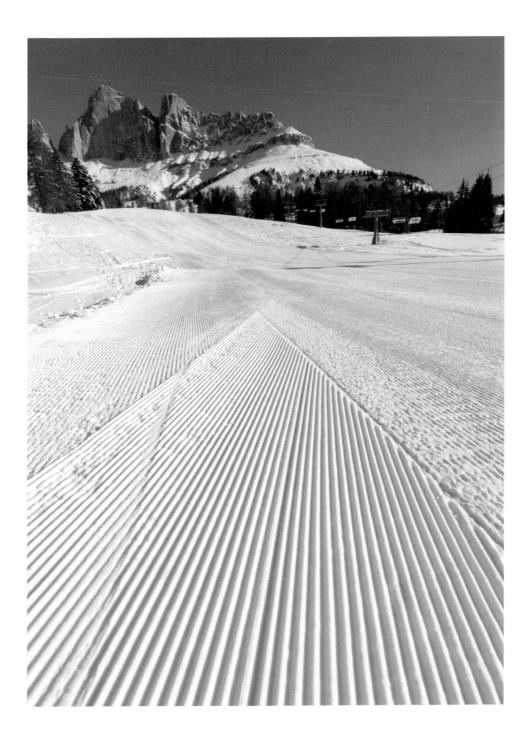

*Morning corduroy is should be pursued like shoppers on "Black Friday" after Thanksgiving
Day as the store doors are opening.*

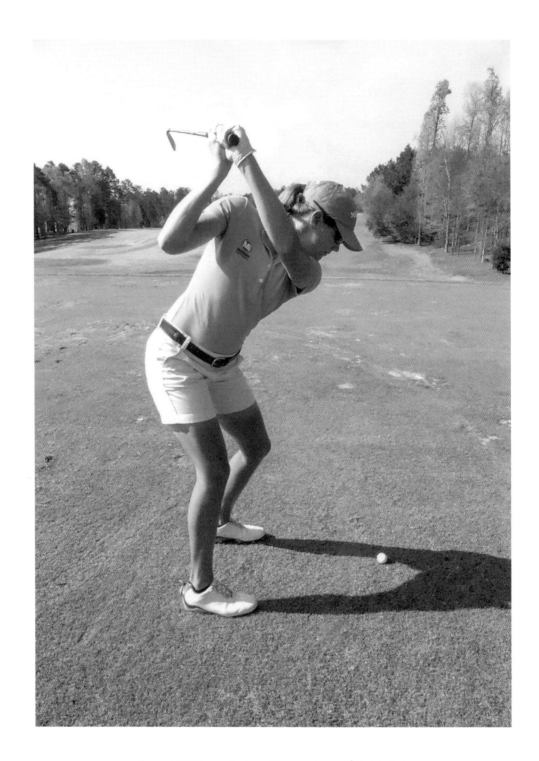

Current LPGA pro, Cydney Clanton, is correctly loaded.

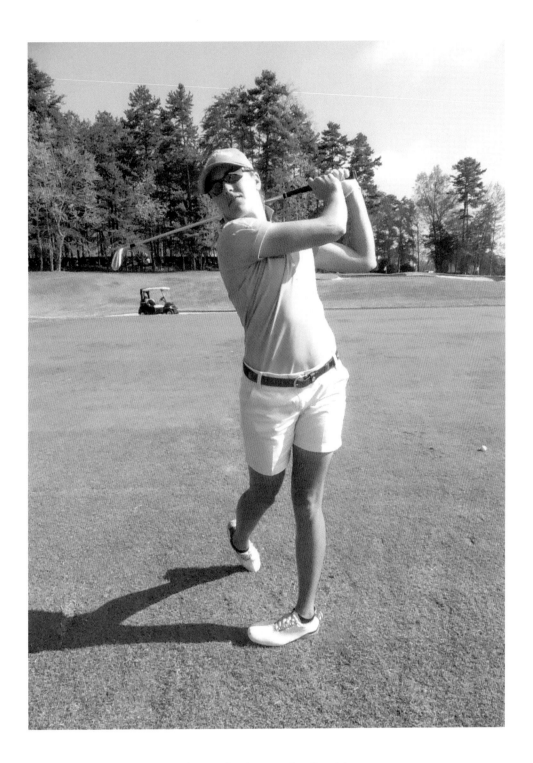

Cydney makes her usual textbook turn.

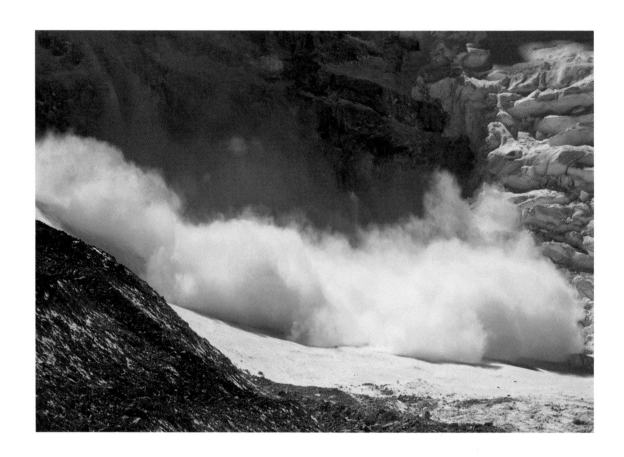

Avalanche Encounter. Four of us were skiing at First (pronounced Furst). We had just gotten off the lift at the very top. About fifty feet past the lift was a glacier- carved 2,500 foot cliff. As we were getting ready to ski we felt what we thought was a earthquake. After a few seconds we realized it was an avalanche; I yelled, "Go!" Twenty or so seconds later, we determined that the avalanche was actually below instead of above us. Interestingly, the bottom of that run ends in the middle of the shopping district in downtown Grindelwald, Switzerland.

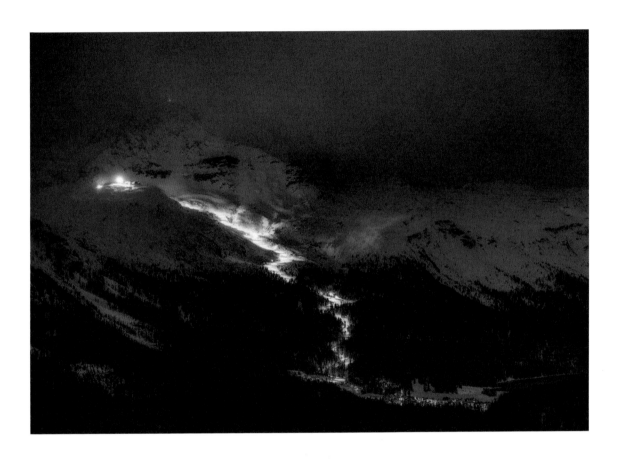

Nothing is as fun as a perfect blue bird ski day but did you know that you can see details in the snow better on a well illuminated ski slope at night? You can see better than on a flat light day or even a very bright sunny day? It's true. Actually, the most fun is skiing with the light of a full moon. It's actually easy. You just aim for the white areas and avoid any dark spots. However, if the dark spot moves or growls, then things may get interesting very fast.

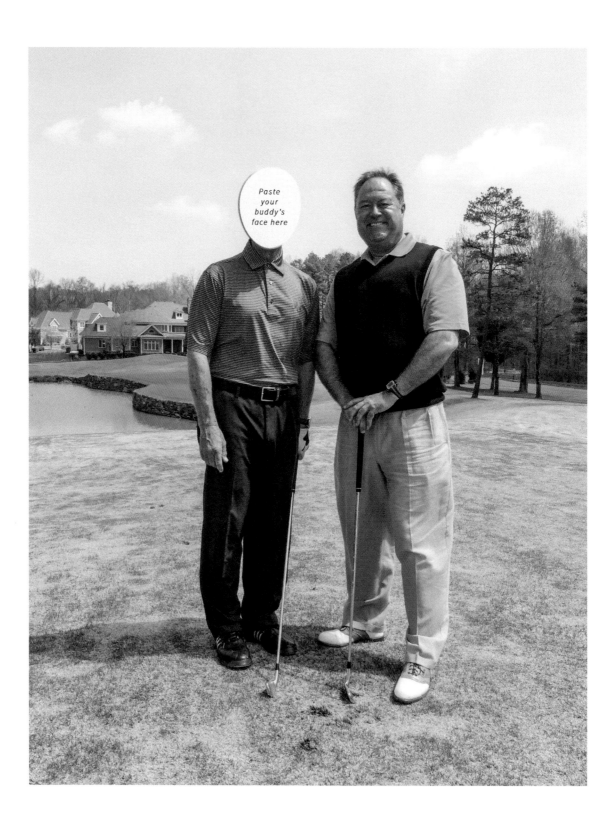

As a yearly tradition, my cousin's wife cuts out and makes a small pile of pictures of her and her friends' faces. She and her circle of friends have such a great time every year pasting pictures of their faces on the pictures of the models in her yearly magazine swimsuit edition. So many heartfelt laughs were created that all agree it is very much worth the time and effort. It turns out those modified magazines are now revered as heirlooms.

So, to refocus this book back on you and your memoires, I recommend and invite you to paste a picture of your best golf or skiing buddy in the white space in the picture to the left to personalize this book for you. Why? This book is intended to rekindle fond memories for you, your friends and family. It will be a fun conversation starter for years to come on your coffee table, for holidays or at parties. Fun will be had by all because everyone wants to talk about their favorite golfing and skiing hero moments.

Better yet, if you want to paste your picture over my face, I'm sure it would be a dramatic improvement! Make yourself or you loved ones look even better. There are plenty of pictures of world-class athletes with perfect form in this book that you may want to personalize. After all, it's your book.

If you're proud of your work, email photos of your pages to mike@golfersandskiers.com and I will put your creativity on my website on the "Wall of Fame" page.

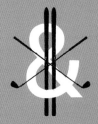

PART III:

THE NUTS AND BOLTS OF TECHNIQUE

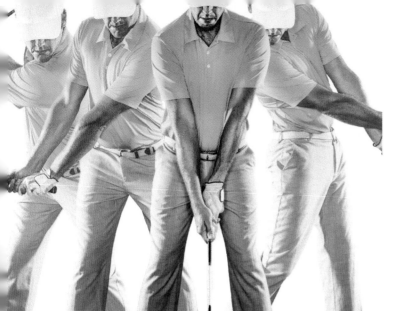
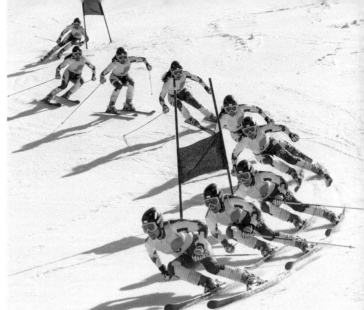

The Sequence

The golf swing is a sequence and a progression of moves. The pivot in the back swing, which many instructors believe is the key move, begins to load the muscles and legs like a stretched rubber band. Once fully loaded, you then release the energy by shifting your weight onto your front leg and rotating your hips towards the target. The upper torso follows the lower body motion by rotating towards the target in a very well timed and sequenced fashion. Your arms, supple wrists and hands maintain a light grip pressure holding the golf club as it swings with increasing speed. The rational swing path of the club approaches the ball with high speed creating a clean strike on the ball with high energy. This is also how a correct skiing turn is made.

In a skiing turn you also load up your abdominal muscles when you finish a turn in preparation for the next, nearly exactly like in a golf turn. Instead of a back swing in golf, in skiing you load up energy by adding pressure on it and standing hard on the outside ski while your shoulders and head face the direction you are going.
As your turn starts, the torque in your abdominals starts to unwind like a rubber band, resulting in your skis being pulled back towards the fall line. When your skis are straight down the hill your edge angle and momentum keep them curving to complete the turn. The effect of your skis now going to the other side of your body again builds torque like a twisted rubber band in your abs in preparation for the next turn.

My most memorable golf spectator experience was being in the stands getting to watch the back-to-back holes in one at Augusta in 2004. Padraig Harrington had a hole in one on Sunday on number 16. Kirk Triplett was about 80 yards away on the 15th green with a clear view of the 16th putting surface when it happened. Kirk put it in the hole from the tee about ten minutes later. The stands erupted in pure joy on both shots.

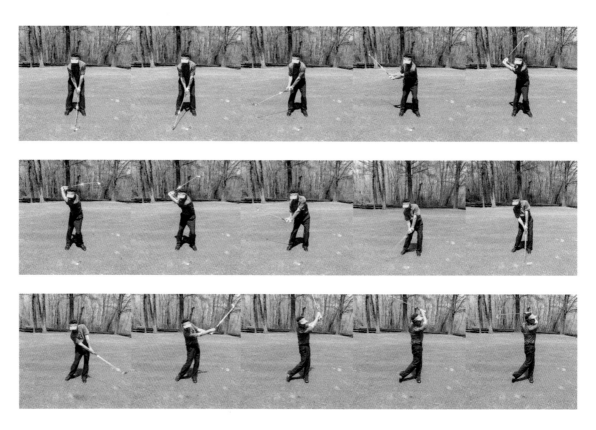

David Ross making a perfect golf stroke.

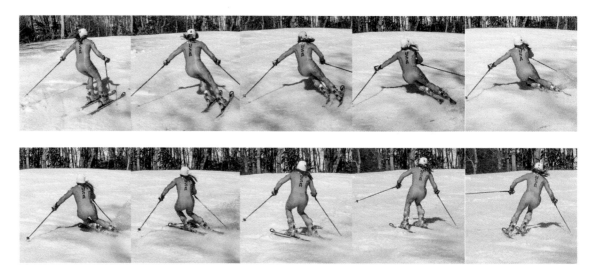

Sarah making a perfect ski turn.

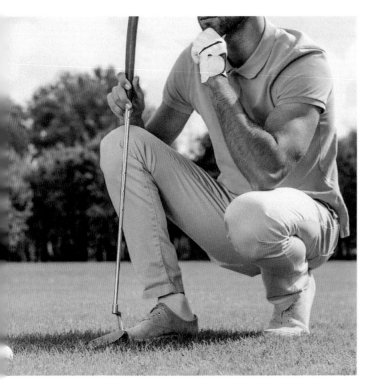 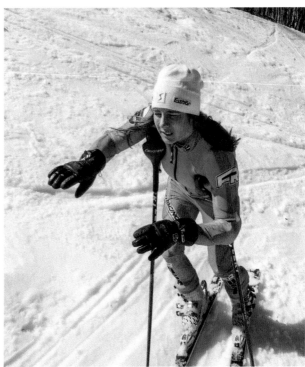

Zen is In. Visualize your plan.

Look at your target and plan your strategy. In golf, you focus on your target and consider the location where you want your ball to land. When playing an approach shot to the green, careful consideration is used, with the golfer focused on the area of the green where they want to ball to land and stop. You need to consider several things like the wind, the length of the grass and hazards before choosing landing sites that increase your chance of success if your shot is not perfect. A proper pre-shot routine includes picking your target, proper alignment to your target and visualizing your shot. The final step in your pre-shot routine should be to ….. relax.

In skiing and ski racing, concentrate on the rise-line and pick a spot above the apex of the turn, or above the gate for the maximum pressure of the turn. In extreme skiing, you need to have a Plan "A", a Plan "B" and a Plan "C". Plan A works if everything goes according to plan. Plan B is in effect if you hit an unexpected rock or miss a turn; what your alternate line must be to get you down with reduced risk. An example of a Plan C may be something like, "If I fall, or do a controlled fall, where would be the best or worst place to land?"

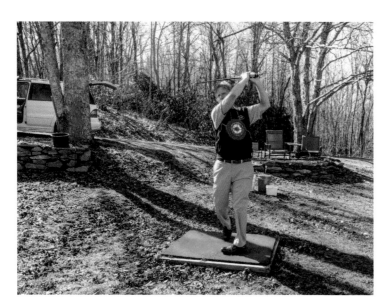
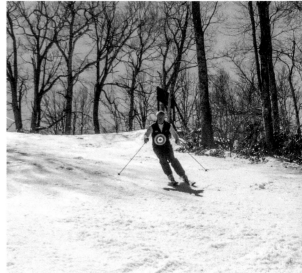

The Belly Button Effect

Proper body rotation and follow-through in golf, as most pros say, is to finish with your belly button facing your target. By creating a strong base with your lower body, you create torque by rotating your shoulders against the resistance of the lower body and core.

Conversely, by ineffectively not using your core you will compensate with your arms or other negative movements resulting in: slices, hooks, fat hits, thin strikes, over-hitting, worm burners, shanks, hitting behind the ball, topping the ball, thrown clubs, broken clubs, a bad attitude and, of course, regrettable language. When you finish the golf stroke with your belly button facing your target, you get a "well done" from your partner and a casual ride in the cart to the middle of the fairway.

When skiing bumps in a slalom of perfect powder or crud, your belly button is also facing your target. In both sports, when you do this, you are in perfect balance and maximizing your bio-mechanical power.

Not to put too fine a point on it, I contend that keeping your belly button lined up is just as important to high-level skiing as to golf, but for polar opposite reasons. In golf, you make the pivot with your hips and core to "load up" the tension like a rubber band, allowing pressure to gather on your solidly planted golf shoe spikes. As your spikes grip the ground, the stored energy is released into the back of the ball. The proper release of this coil turns your shoulders faster, thereby providing the power your arms and wrists generate to control club head speed.

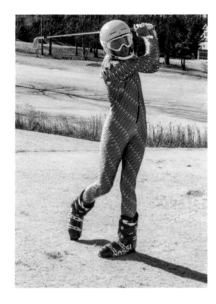 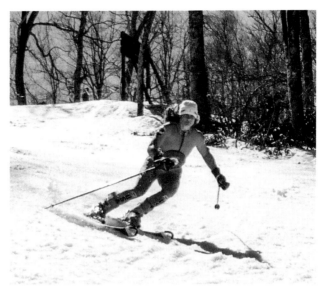

*(Left)
Cydney is one of
the best female
golfers in the
world.*

*(Right)
Sarah is one of the
best female skiers
in the world.*

In snow skiing, skiing bumps, skiing through trees, skiing crud, and specifically slalom racing, it is the polar opposite, because your shoulders are the part of your body that stays one hundred percent still. However, your core is just as torqued as in a golf swing. In skiing, the core is torqued to help the legs and feet receive the pent-up core energy. The more the belly button faces the direction of where you want to go, the more energy you will have in your feet and skis to bring them around with controlled power for a smooth and powerful ski turn.

The ending position should be with your feet firmly anchored to the ground while your shoulders act as a fulcrum. Conversely, in skiing, your shoulders are the constant or stationary body-part, while your legs and feet are the fulcrum. However, in both sports the middle is your core. To get the maximum controllable energy in the torqued core like a rubber band, you need to keep your belly button facing your target.

- In golf, the energy is created in the golfer's core between the shoulders and the hips.
- In skiing, the twist point between the legs and the hips with the torque still stored in the core.
- However, the end result is the same position per the pictures above.

In conclusion, in golf , your feet are stationary and your shoulders move. In skiing, you shoulders are stationary and your lower body and feet move.

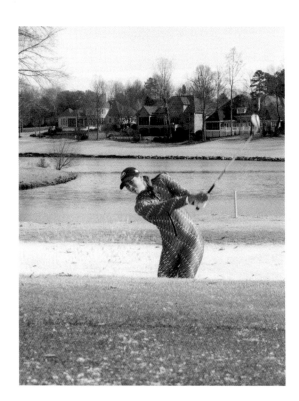 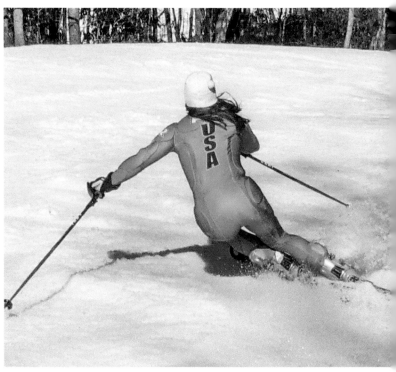

The Body "C"

The correct form for power and accuracy in both sports comes down to the letter "C". When you put your body in a power "C" position your hip muscles, abs and legs can produce the explosive power needed for a high speed ski turn or the ability to hit a ball with energy and timing. In addition to power generation, the opening of the hips releases the legs to work independently. In golf, this allows the legs to create power with the weight shift and un-twisting of the abs and back. The momentum lets the arms and wrist whip around for controlled greater club head speed. The "C" helps the skier roll onto the edges or increased edge angle increasing the curve and reducing the skid for a smooth and powerful turn. Like a race car on a banked turn or a motocross racer on a berm, the skier can then put more centrifugal force onto the heavily angled ski edge with less chance of it sliding out. When a skier's ski slides out, pressure on the ski to make it bend is less and the result is lost speed, lost smoothness and lost power.

In ski racing you should always have a plan at the start of your run, a common strategic plan for many is, "flash or crash." - Anonymous

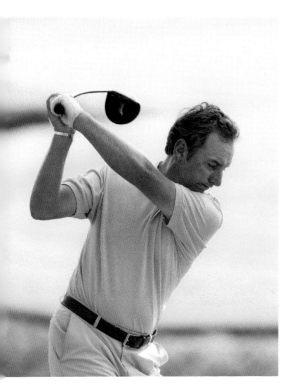
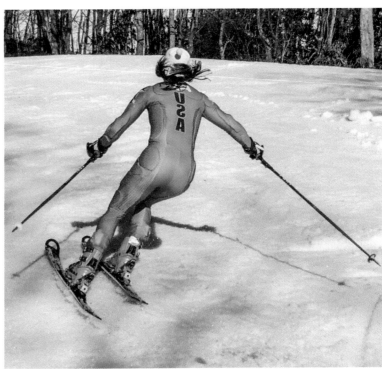

Bending metal is the goal

In skiing and in golf, the interim goal is bending metal or carbon fiber. In skiing, what you can control is how you bend the ski on edge. High-level skiers use the ski as a tool. How and where they bend it shapes the turn, controls their speed and they either arc or slide to the desired direction or spot for the next turn. The skier's skills to bend the ski combined with the physical attributes of the ski are the determining factors. Likewise, the golfer's skill-level and the physical characteristics of the golf club shaft greatly impact the direction of the ball trajectory. In both sports, the rebound of the metal, wood, or carbon fiber amplifies the power and speed of the turn and the club head speed of the golf swing. Your ability to maximize the bend and the rebound of the materials is in direct correlation to your success in both sports at advanced and expert levels.

All golfers know, "it just takes one good shot to bring you back" – Anonymous.

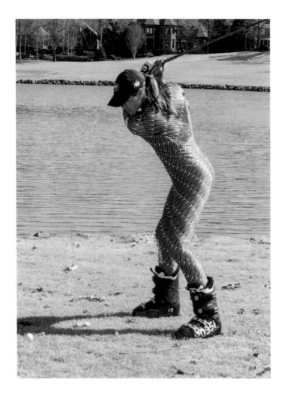 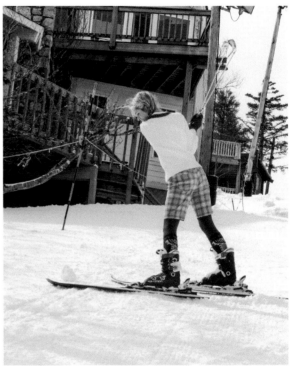

Slow and early

Begin the backswing slowly. Slight pressure starts to build very early in the golf turn as the shoulders rotate. As the blade of the golf club begins to rotate, torque builds in the golfer's waist. At the completion of the backswing, the pressure is released in a controlled explosion of energy. Torque builds in the midsection of skiers in almost exactly the same way. As the skier keeps the body facing downhill, torque builds while the skis jet from one turn to the other. As the skis jet well past under the center of mass, the torque increases as the edge pressure decreases while the skis begin to roll to the other edge. Similarly, the backswing in golf is wound up as far as it will go until the release forces a change of direction of the club head. In a similar manner the torso tension starts the ski change of direction by unwinding in a dynamic and powerful way.

As the golf swing begins and proceeds to the midpoint, the shaft is bent to provide extra whip on the ball. The ski is also bent to the maximum at the midpoint of the arch of the turn to provide kinetic energy to propel the skier or racer in a smooth but powerful release of energy. Some golf shafts are more flexible, just as some skis are more flexible. The more advanced shafts for pros and people who swing hard are stiffer. Just as with golf shafts, expert- level and racing skis are stiffer and require much more energy than softer skis. Both skis and golf clubs are made with titanium, graphite composite, fiber, plastic and even wood. In both sports, a slow, relatively gradual bend is usually best. Ted Ligety starts his turn slower and earlier than any of his competitors on the tour. With the change in equipment, regulations restricting parabolic racing skis to the old straight design, Ligety's dominance in the giant slalom altered, as the technology was reduced at the highest level.

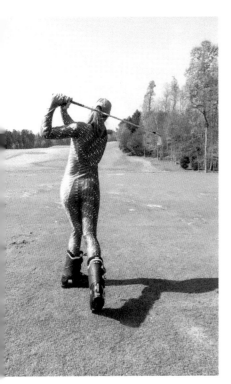 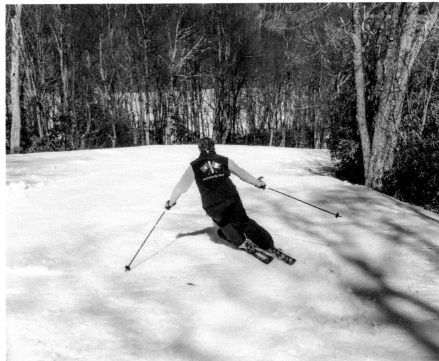

Completion and follow-through

In both golfing and skiing, the finish is critical. In a golf swing, the biomechanics of the follow-through is just as important as the rest of the stroke. The follow-though directs the aim and tempo of the swing. If you consider the start of the arc of the swing plane as point "A" and the end of the swing as point "B", you want a smooth club swing on the arc for accuracy and distance. Golfers have heard-- and most have also said-- "One good swing will bring you back." We all know this to be true. One good run or shot will bring you back.

In skiing, the "completion of the turn" controls the skier's speed and is therefore biomechanically critical for the next linked turn. As the skis start the turn in the part of the turn before the skis have reached directly downhill, the skier's weight has already been placed on the outside ski. You begin to ride a smooth edge in an arc as the pressure on the outside ski increases. At the bottom of the turn when your downhill boot and ski are below you, you let the ski continue to track in front of your body with your legs moving in a pendulum motion as your body is falling forward. When your skis jet past your body, it is called "completing the turn". The reason this is important is that you want your skis as far as you can on the other side of your body to have a step edge angle as you start to pressure your outside edge to counter the centrifugal force on your new ski edge.

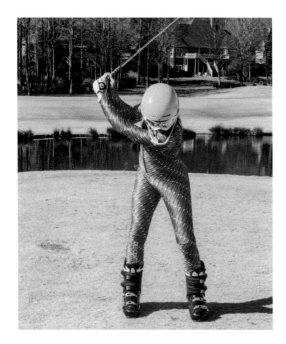 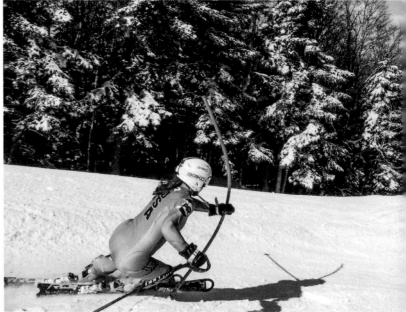

Heads!!!

In both golfing and skiing the head should not move; not at all. Some golf pros have variations on head movement or placement, but by and large, your head should be a constant or non-variable in a good golf swing. A quiet head helps keep the swing plane consistent. A stationary head acts as a starting point of the swing plane helping remove unwanted swing flaws. Most importantly, a steady head position helps the golfer swing the club back squarely impact, consistently striking the ball in the sweet spot. Masters Champion Jordan Speith, is the prime example of a golfer who keeps his head perfectly still.

Moreover, in skiing moguls either for fun or competition, skiers are told to pretend there is a wire going from the top of the slope to the bottom of the slope. You want that wire to go through your head all the way down the run. Zero head movement makes all the difference in the position of your core, hips, knees, ankles and feet, as the effect of the energy to be released. In other words, your head should not move at all the whole way down the slope. Zero up and down and zero side to side. This concept clearly translates to all good skiing turns and golf swings.

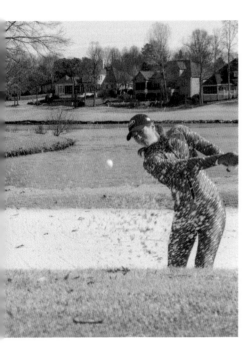 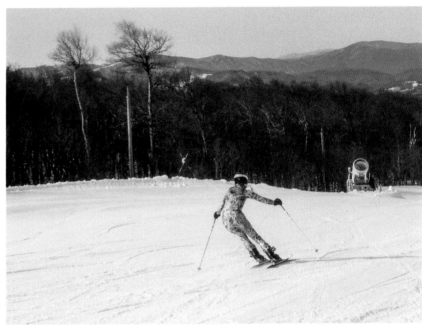

Arms are OUT and hips are IN for golf and skiing

Both golfing and skiing get the vast majority of their power from the legs, abdomen, back, ankles and hips. In golf, your power is from your legs and hips and the torque of your lower body. The same is true for skiing. In both sports, the hands lightly hold the golf club or ski poles just enough so the poles or clubs do not come out of your hands. The dichotomy of intense lower-body, core torque, loose upper-body and zero head movement are unique to only golf and skiing. Rework this. Arms remain fairly connected to the torso in golf. Arms are away from the torso in skiing, but equally uninvolved in the turn.

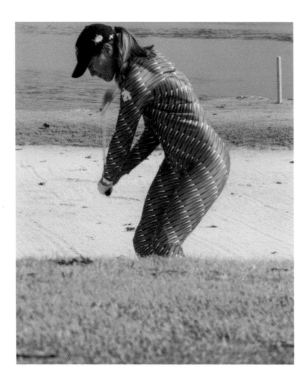 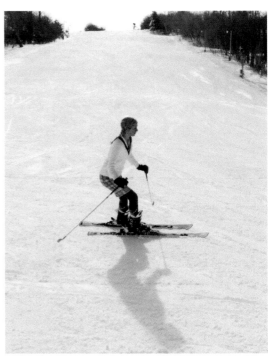

Loose Wrists and Arms

The name of the game for both amateurs and pros is to maximize their distance on the golf course by swinging smoothly, which results in faster club head speed. If your arms and wrists are tight, it may be bio-mechanically impossible to get the maximum whip through impact. If you are tight, tired, or stiff in your arms and wrists, it is hard to increase the club head speed for power and is disruptive to swinging through the ball correctly. If your grip pressure is light and your wrists and arms are supple, you can smoothly create good tempo, timing and club head speed for longer, more accurate and more controlled shots. Remember, in golf, the power is generated via the trunk and torso, but it is released though impact by soft, released arms and hands. Hence, your arms are just along for the ride and as a guide for your hands.

Interestingly enough, skiing is the same. The only part of your upper body that is supposed to move is your wrists. Moreover, your wrists need to be relaxed just like in a proper golf stroke. In addition, like in golf, any other upper body movement is counterproductive causing bad things to happen. In skiing, you want steady arms and loose wrists help with proper biomechanical body position, balance and improved timing. It is counter-intuitive, but relaxed wrists are critical for bump skiing and skiing through trees. Also, like golf, the whole ski turn is done with the lower body and core.

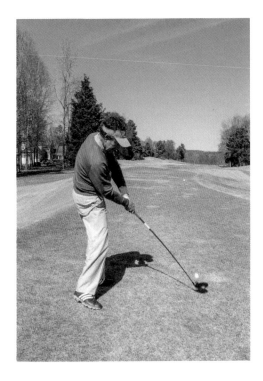 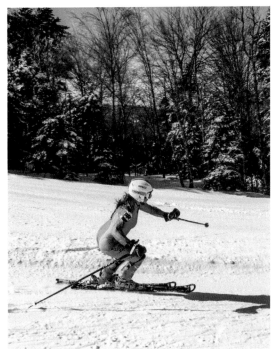

(Left) David is loaded up.

(Right) Sarah's ski is loaded and bent.

The pre-apex and finish of the arc is central to skiing and golf

In golf, it is called the smooth backswing. In skiing, it is called starting your turn early. I have always humorously said I should be a great golfer, since my backswing is faster than all the pros on the circuit. That begs the rhetorical question, how's that working out for me so far? The reason Ted Ligety skis giant slalom better than anyone in the history of skiing is because he starts his turns and presses on his skis earlier than any other top-level racer in the world. Hence, he starts his pre-arc earlier resulting in a smoother, rounder and faster turn. To see an example, do a Google search on "Ted Ligety arcs" and watch some videos. However, what about his "big skid" that helped him win the gold medal in the 2014 Olympics? Yes, Ted did do a huge tactical skid called a skivot (skid/pivot) at a particularly hard gate that was fraught with disaster. However, remember he had a two full-second lead over the field before the start of his last run. The skid cost him 1.5 seconds, but he had a half-second to spare. Smart tactical move.

When learning to ski off-piste with my buddy Patrick Rothe, when we came up to a cliff or hidden drop-off, he would always say, "It's probably not all that steep over there." … and I would follow him.

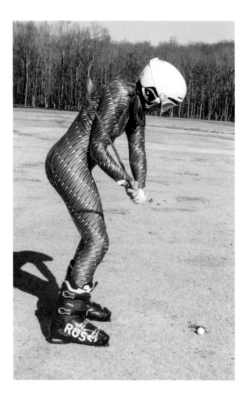

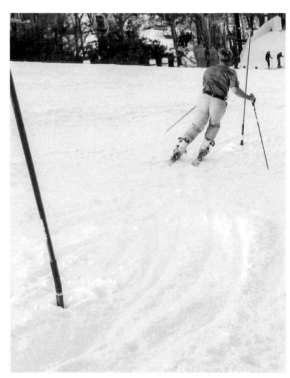

(Left)
Cydney near max energy in her down stroke.

(Right)
Jason is past max pressure above the gate. Like most skiers, if you normally start your turn here, you are far too late.

70% of the swing or turn energy is expended before the apex of the arc

The point of impact is clearly where the rubber meets the road in golf. After the ball has been struck, the player does not have any control over the ball. To the chagrin of many, it can be proven that talking to the ball or engaging body English after the ball is in the air or rolling, really does not help. This is obvious in golf. You have the long backswing and the downward energy to the bottom of the arc where contact is made. But in skiing, energy expended above the apex of the turn is less obvious and seldom done even though it is just as important. By the apex of the turn, your skis should be facing down the fall line or straight downhill. To make the ski work for you correctly, you need to pressure the outside ski when it is going in the "wrong" direction of the way you want to go.

This sounds strange and feels even stranger, but it is vital to a correct ski turn. If you do not start the turn before your skis have drifted to the fall line, you will have lost all your core torque and all you can really achieve is a bouncy, skidding turn. Skid-turns can only be done on groomed or icy slopes. In powder, heavy snow, off-piste, in the trees, or some wet snow conditions, you are out of luck and will be exhausted in a few runs. That is why most people like groomed runs, so they can make do with their less than ideal technique. It actually takes far more effort to ski incorrectly than correctly. When you ski correctly, your skis do most of the work and you just ride them. When you ski incorrectly, you push snow instead of riding it. One of my biggest learning moments in skiing was when an Olympic racer announced to a crowd of amateurs that, "Seventy percent of your energy needs to be expended above the gate." Unlike watching Slammin' Sam Sneed, this sunk in and I won an amateur national title. I just stood on my outside ski as soon as I could and I was much smoother and faster.

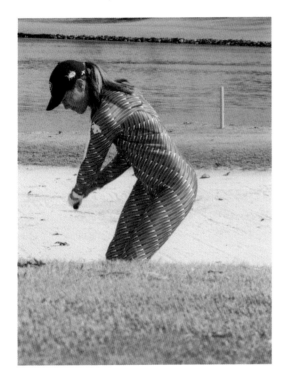 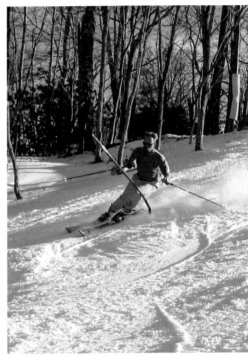

(Left) Cydney nearing max club head speed.

(Right) Jason taking one on the knee for your benefit in his seersucker pants and golf shirt.

The Maximum Energy Point

In golf it is all about making solid contact with the ball. All the tips and tactics in this book, and all the others that you have read, lead up to the point of ball contact. It is like driving a high- performance sports car like a Porsche or a Formula One race car; All the road sees are the tires. Everything else above the tires in a car is to support the tire/road contact. All the golf equipment and body movements are in support of that point of contact between the club face and the golf ball. After the apex or contact point momentum moves the hands, shoulders, and golf club through the rest of the plane of the swing, the biomechanics cause a stopping point of the golf swing which is called "follow through".

The apex of the ski turn is the point when the most pressure is applied to the outside foot and front of the ski boot. That energy is transmitted through the riser and bindings to the ski. Your energy from your foot causes the ski to bend for a smooth carved turn. As seen in the skiing sequence pictures in the "Sequence Chapter", the pressure is reduced as you begin to transition to the new ski for your next ski turn.

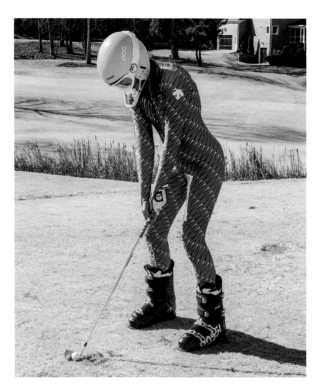 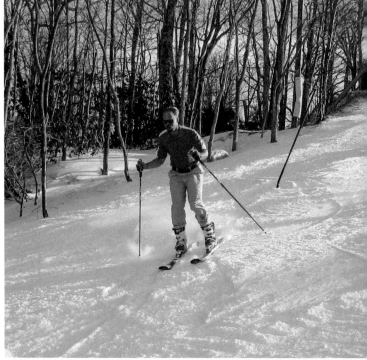

Balance

In most sports, the better balance you have the better you will perform. Almost all sports start in an athletic and balanced stance. The good news is that the perfect athletic balanced stance is the same in golfing and skiing. Have your feet shoulder-width apart, your hands out in front and your knees slightly bent. That is the same starting stance for golf, skiing, tennis, baseball, most football positions and basketball. If you start in that stance, you will be in the same starting position as the current and active pros. After that, the amateurs digress. Maintaining proper and needed balance in most all sports, including golf and skiing, once you start moving, comes from proper and correct biomechanical movement.

"In a balanced and athletic stance, you could ski down any mountain in the world… You just may not be able to stop." says my skiing mentor Jim Cottrell.

If a golfer loses his or her balance during a swing, the ball could miss the target by a few yards. Another outcome could be the sound of breaking glass. Even worse balance will result in a fall. Worst of all is if someone takes a video of the fall or the breaking glass. Bad balance in skiing can have even more dire negative reinforcement. A face plant, crashing into your buddy, or hitting something that does not move are key reasons to keep your balance.

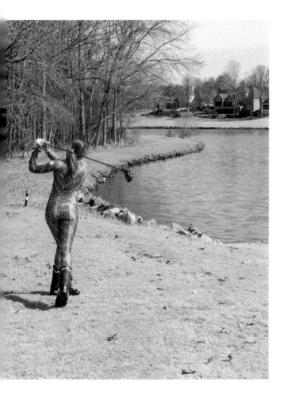 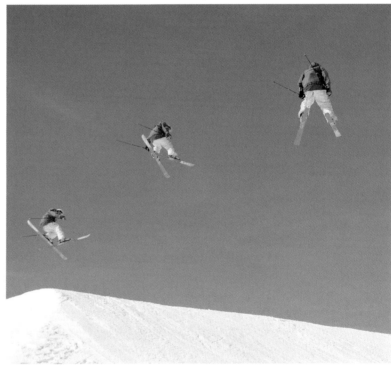

Golf and skiing require far more athleticism than is advertised

 I'm tired of hearing people say on the radio and other media that, "Golf is not a sport."! My reply to them is:

Most baseball players get a home run if they hit a ball 300 feet. To me, that's just a 9 iron distance. Wake me up when they can hit a ball over 1,000 feet like an amateur golfer.

We think a professional baseball player is great if he can throw a ball 100 miles an hour. When a good amateur golfer hits a drive, it leaves the tee box at 180 mph.

Ski racers reach up to a G-Force of 3.5. That means a 200 pound man will need to control 700 pounds of pressure on his legs while making turns on ice and snow at speeds of over 80 miles per hour. In the TV show The SuperStars, high-profile professional athletes are pitted against each other. Snow skiers beat out all the other football, baseball, basketball, soccer and tennis Olympians for the last three years of the show. Some other examples include the following:

> In 2001, former Austrian brick layer-turned-world champion ski racer, Herrman Maier (The Herrmanator) won the Super Stars Championship on the TV series. He beat out all the star professional football players, basketball players, soccer players in that competition in the obstacle course that year.

> In 2002, Bode Miller shattered the obstacle course record for the multi-year duration of the show by not using the rope to climb the nine-foot-tall wooden wall. Instead, using his mountain climbing techniques, he jumped and grabbed the top of the wall with his fingertips and hurdled the wall in one smooth motion. During that season, his training technique of pulling his family's lawn tractor on a gravel road with just a harness left many watchers, including me, in awe.

> The all-time reigning Super Stars champion from the TV series is free-style skier Jeremy Bloom. So why is Jeremy the reigning champion, you ask? Because the program was canceled after he won. I would surmise that the producers of the show would have preferred the latest NFL star be crowned the champion for ratings reasons. However, as a biased skier and golfer, I would say… "Scoreboard."

So, when people chuckle at snow skiers or golfers being athletes, I bring up these facts and say: "Scoreboard."

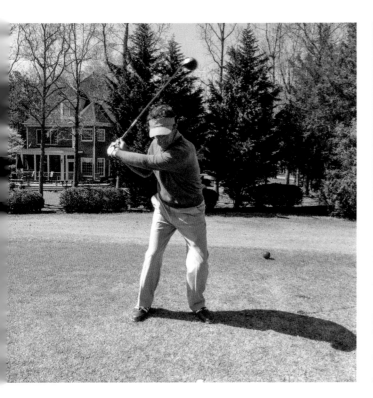 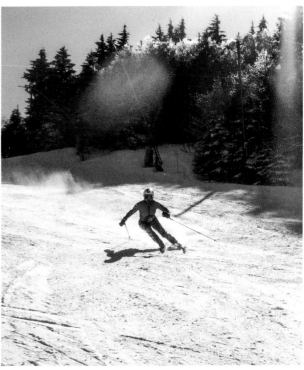

Swing on Plane and the Perfect Arc in the Snow

Both sports rely heavily on biomechanics, physics, and timing. To compound the problem, both sports require you to complete your tasks in three-dimensional space. In golf, you have to use the coiling of the body to release and get the club face to return to the exact same spot to strike the ball correctly. To do that, you need to be on a two-dimensional plane. The fact that golf is played, and skiing is performed, on uneven terrain further complicates things. In other words, in both sports you have to make a two-dimensional swing or round turn with the added dimension of an uneven surface resulting in a three-dimensional aspect in both sports. Bowling and tennis would be an examples of a two-dimensional sports. The extra dimensions cause more difficulty, challenge, interest and fascination resulting in the popularity and devotion to our sports.

The obvious example in skiing is taking a mogul run or bump run. You are clearly working in a three-definitional situation that is moving as well. You want your feet to be in soft constant contact with the snow regardless of differences in the terrain, as well as constant turning to control your speed.

The perfect golf swing needs to be on plane. Bad things happen when you are swinging off-plane. Topped balls, worm burners, hits too far behind the ball, hooks, duck hooks, slices, and lost golf balls are just several of disasters that happen. (A duck hook is when you hook the ball and yell – "duck".) An on-plane swing yields a controlled shot that finds fairways most of the time, or comes to rest on the green near the flag.

A controlled shot that is on plane has a better chance to hit the fairway, the green, or your target. Moreover, when your swings are on plane, you can begin to introduce spin, or shaping to your shots. To draw the ball for a dog-leg left or for more roll, you can change your plane up or down. To fade the ball, you make your plane slightly more vertical. If you are confused and not normal because you hit the ball from the wrong side I cannot help that, lefties.

Like golf, in skiing the goal of any intermediate or advanced skier to make a perfect arced turn is by leaving railroad track marks in the snow. The objective is to leave two pencil thin edge marks in the snow with zero skid. This is evidence of a perfectly carved turn with power, control, speed and balance. To make "railroad tracks" in the snow, lean forward to start the turn so you put pressure on the ski tips and they will dig into the snow. Then, roll the ankles to increase the edge angle so the ski can bend and track evenly. And finally, fully complete the turn by letting the skis move past your body as they transition to the next turn. Most people can get the rolling the skis on edges part. The new technology of shaped skies rewards skiers that do this. Fewer can complete the turn fully. Even fewer start their turn early enough on a consistent basis. Practice linking complete turns together on the easy groomers but at speed so you can stay stable and have enough force to bend the ski. After some practice, then try the steeper groomers and see if you can make two pencil-thin railroad tracks in the snow with your ski edges like the pros.

Weight Back Equals Disaster

In golf, when your weight is on your back foot, especially at the end of your finish, it is usually a disastrous shot. Other than a few high-risk rescue shots, hitting the ball with your weight back results in all kinds of bad results. Topping the ball, hitting fat, slice, hook, worm burners, fits of anger, extreme frustration and grounding the club are just some of the outcomes of finishing with your weight on your back foot. When your weight is moving forward towards your front leg, your swing will produce a stroke with more control, more distance and the desired shape and spin are greatly improved. At the top of the backswing with an iron, the weight should be distributed slightly more on the back foot. With a longer club, like a driver, approximately 80% of the weight should gather on the back foot. The down-swing starts the lateral shift of the weight towards the front leg.

Weight on your heels is as bad for recreational skiers as for golfers and will eventually result in potentially painful crashes for racers, bump skiers and tree skiers. The golf stroke and optimum ski turn differ in the fact that in golf, the player moves from neutral to forward, while skiers should move far forward to initiate the turn then ease back towards neutral as they reach full weight on the downhill ski in the apex of the turn. This may seem odd to most until you remember that the full weight forward is to initiate the turn. To push your weight forward you must, at some point, ease-off to have room to move forward again. Moreover, when I say move forward, I recommend that you move forward breaking with your ankles and ABSOLUTLY NOT AT YOUR WAIST. Most all beginners break at the waist, which is counterproductive; an unintended consequence of moving your "rear end" on the back of your skis. You are better off staying neutral and not moving at all than bending at your waist. The reason for the full-body lean at your ankles is to put pressure on the very front edge of your ski. This pressure will make that part of the ski dig into the snow to start the ski to bend from the tip. This called "hooking up the tips" and is exactly what you want to happen. It is so much fun to do when you get it down because it makes the ski do the work resulting in the start of a perfectly carved turn. In addition, it puts your body weight over your bones, not on your quads to further save your energy and effort. Golf is very similar. You want to stack over your turn with no waist bend. If you bend at the waist you cannot make a smooth turn on the ball.

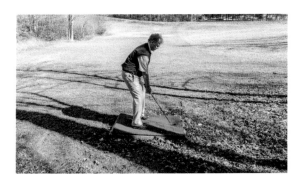
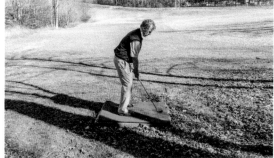

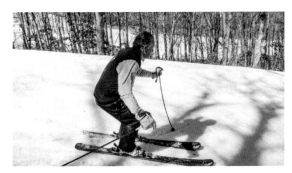
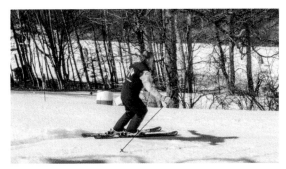

Jim with weight on his heels.   *Jim with correct weight distribution.*

Situational Tactics

By design, good golf courses test your skills by forcing you to hit a variety of different shots. The standard and most practiced shots are below.

- The drive with a driver or three wood.
- The long iron with a two through four iron.
- The approach shot with a five iron to the pitching wedge.
- The sand shot with your sand wedge.
- The chip lofted with an iron or edge.
- The long and short putt with your putter.

But what happens when things do not go exactly as planned? If you have to hit from under a tree; you have an extreme side hill lie; there is a tree between you and the green; or you have to hit over a bunker with little green to work with, what do you do? Now things get interesting. You are going to have to use a situational shot or tactic. Practice these shots and you will gain confidence and reduce your score average. I recommend you consider spending practice time on the following situational shots that are occasionally needed:

The knock down shot is a shot hit back in the stance to keep it low. It is used when under a tree or on a high wind day.

The fade shot is used to bend the shape of the shot trajectory from left to right for right handed players, the fade used to curve the ball around a dog leg right hole or to spin the ball to the right on the approach to the green; this is done by changing the arc of the swing or the grip.

The draw shot is the converse of the fade. Moreover, the draw shot bends the shape of the ball trajectory to the left for right-handed players. Since the ball has a lower trajectory, the ball will roll out for added distance.

The flop shot is played with a sand wedge, which has the most loft of all the clubs, and is played when you are trying to go over sand or other hazard and need to stop the ball with as little roll as possible. This shot should be used as a last resort option by most golfers.

The bump and run is used to bounce the ball onto the green as a safe option; one could consider this shot to be a shorter version of the knockdown shot since it is usually hit from back in the stance. The key to the bump and run is picking the target of the first bounce and speed control.

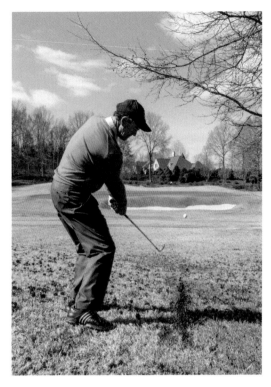

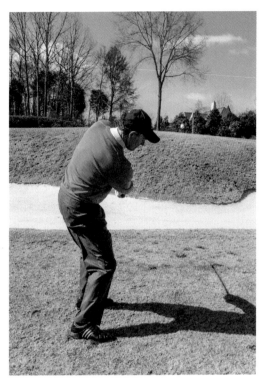

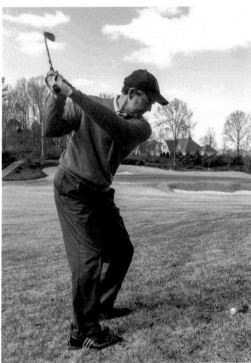

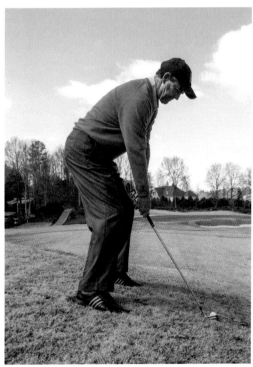

(Top Left)
Perfectly executed
knockdown shot.
(missed by 18
inches)

(Top Right)
Flop shot by
David Ross,
PGA Professional.

(Bottom Left)
Side hill above
the feet.

(Bottom Right)
Side hill below
the feet.

High level skiers have just as many kinds of turns to learn to perfect. The difference here is that in high-level skiing, things happen faster and the consequences can be more painful when out-of-the-norm situations develop. Like in golfing, skiing has a baseline of common turns:

The carving turn, the normal racing turn, or turn used on groomers with energy at the top of the turn.

The skidding turn is used by beginners, to reduce speed and primary tactic for bump skiers.

The wedge (snowplow) even used by high level skiers in certain situations.

Short radius turns, are quick turns down the fall line.

Medium or long radius turns, are more elongated arcs in the snow for faster turns or lesser pitched slopes

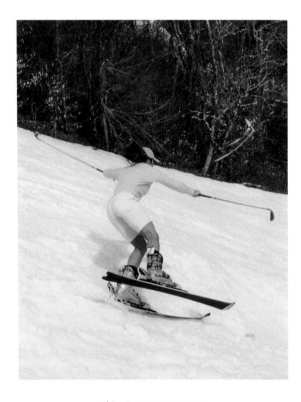

White Pass recovery turn.

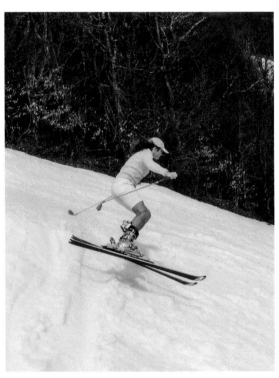

Scoot turn to avoid trouble.

Like in golf, things do not always go as planned, or you approach some terrain where normal turn tactics do not apply. Now you need to draw on your repertoire of turns and tactics. The following is a list of specialty turns and tactics that are useful when the situation arises:

The scoot turn is when you go airborne to avoid a hole, rut, snow snake (stick or rock) or something you just do not want to ski through or over. See Sarah's scoot turn above as she jumps over a hole.

The diverging and converging turn is a turn that is used cut off a turn to miss rock or any object, or to step over a rock.

The White Pass turn is when you start and put all your weight on your inside ski. This is one of the most used recovery turns. The White Pass turn got its name from the White Pass Ski area *www.skiwhitepass.com* where the Mahre brothers perfected this inside ski move to initiate their racing turns. To execute this turn, you begin by leaning your inside knee in as far as you can as your first move in the turn. In the White Pass drill, you only ski on the inside edge for the first half of the turn with your downhill ski staying in the air. Most dramatic downhill ski racing recoveries you see on TV highlights are some form of the White Pass turn. Hence, skiers are highly encouraged to practice skiing on their outside edge as practice. Take a high-level lesson to learn the right way to do this drill. Most ski coaches will have their athletes take one ski off at the top of the run to force them to practice this drill. See Sarah's recovery to the left using a White Pass move.

The skivot turn, skid/pivot, is used when you are sliding on ice, then jam your edges at once into the snow to change your trajectory from a slide to forward. The most famous skivot turn was used by Ted Lighety as a risk-reducing tactic to protect his lead to win one of his Olympic gold medals.

The crud turn uses a fundamentally correct turn in crud snow. Crud snow is defined as cut up powder, heavy wet snow, mash potato snow, snow with an ice layer on top or any other highly variable snow and very steep terrain. The crud turn consists of three moves:
- *Placing your weight on both shins all the time*
- *Fully committing to starting your turn extra early to make full "S" turns*
- *Pretending you are skiing in a culvert that is six inches shorter than you are, thus your head can never hit the top of the culvert.*

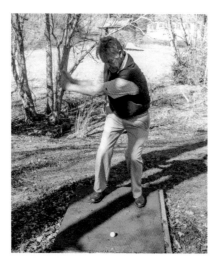 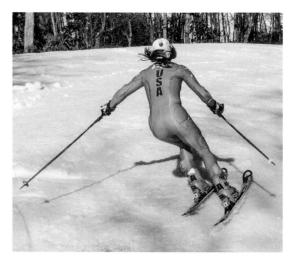

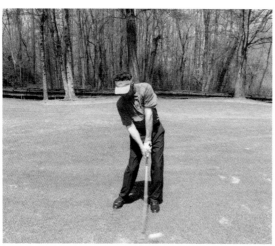 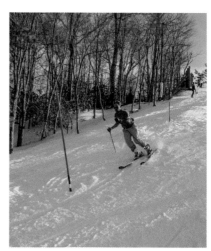

Drive it into the ground

On the golf down-stroke when hitting an iron, you focus on driving the club head into the ground behind the ball. In other words, you want to hit down on the ball. A properly executed downswing with iron will result in the ball being struck with a slightly downward action though the impact area. When the ball is struck with a descending angle, the ball will fly higher resulting from the club head angle. Even better, it will create more backspin to help you control the shape of the flight. You will notice striking the ball this way allows you to properly apply the various lofts of each iron in your bag. Your distance will greatly improve as the result. You will leave a clean divot after the ball is struck. Remembering to repair your divot is good golf etiquette.

The initiation of a correct recreational and racing ski turn is similar. You want to lean forward at your ankles (not at your waist) to drive the side of the tip of your ski into snow to start the ski bending to create the arching bent ski and the smooth and controlled arching turn. Without driving the tip into the snow, there is no way to "hook up" your tips to start a non-skidded turn. Your goal is to have two pencil-thin arcs in the snow from just your ski edges. Just forward knee pressure on your boots is not enough in most cases. You need to lean forward with your body out ahead of your boots at the very beginning of the turn with your upper body AND hips. Bending at the waist to get forward, as intermediates do, is far worse than just staying in a neutral body position. You want to be forward, but thinking you are being safe by being back because the hill is so steep. The bad news is it does not work. With your rear-end back, there is far too much weight on the back of your skis and they will not turn without great effort, and you'll go into a flat skid or a basic snowplow. What you should do is lean forward at your ankles with your whole body about five to ten degrees at the beginning of the turn for a smooth carved turn.

In most ski towns the guy to gal ration is 5:1. The gals say, "The odds are good but the goods are odd." The guys say, "You don't lose your girlfriend, you just lose your turn." - Anonymous

The Future

Intense passion breeds more passion. The future of our sports will be in good hands as parents share their love for our sports with their sons and daughters. You may have been lucky enough to have had many fond memories of time skiing and golfing with your parents or other family members. Your kids, nieces and nephews will have the same warm memories when they are your age. You may be thinking about some of those memories right now. That makes it all worth it.

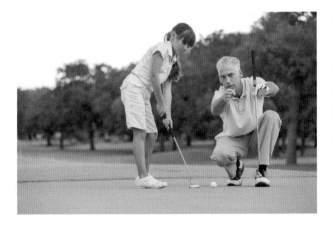
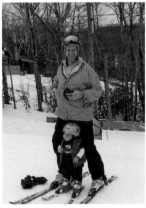

THE END

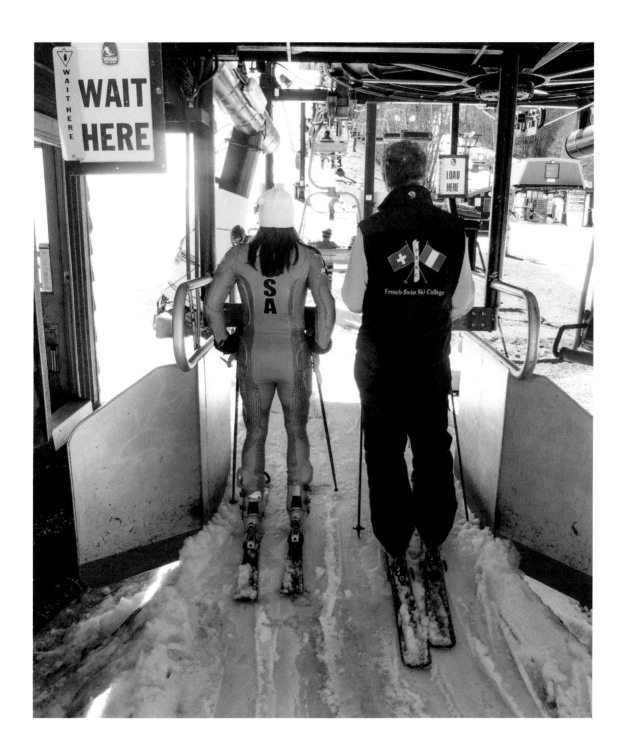

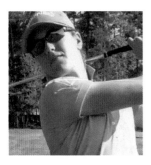

Cydney Clanton – LPGA tour 2013, 2014, 2015. Winner on the Symetra Tour. Curtis Cup Member. World Amateur Team Member. Four time All American at Auburn University. Two time winner as an amateur – Woman's North South Championship and NCAA Fall Preview. Thank you for help with the golfing pictures. I was honored that you would agree to help me. I look forward to following you on the LPGA tour for many years. "As professional athletes as much as we would like to say we got here all by ourselves it tends to not be the case. I have a great support team and truly appreciate all they have done. Thank you to Milksplash, Modern Impressions, JWL 360 project, and Southern Tide."

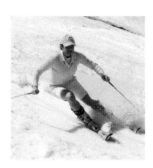

Sarah Dockery Bliss – 2012 Second Fastest Overall US Amateur Female (NASTAR Race of Champions). Full college scholarship for skiing. Has bested many former Olympic alpine racers and former US Team members. Currently, she owns a large scale pet sitting business in the Charlotte area. Thanks for the multiple trips to the mountains for the photo shoots and your friendship.

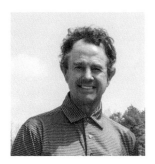

David Ross – is a PGA pro and Director of Golf at River Run County Club in Davidson, NC (Home of the Chiquita Classic). David has coached many successful golfers. David facilitated many of the golfing shots in this book and arranged for me to contact Cydney. His help and friendship were invaluable to the creation of *Golfers & Skiers*. I hope you find many helpful insights to help your golf game in this book. Many of the best points were clarified and refocused by David. He is a pros pro. There is no way to thank you enough. Moreover, David coached, and still coaches, Cydney since she was a little girl. Now she is one of the best female golfers in the world. If your phenom needs some extra help, you may want to contact David at dross@riverruncc.com. See Cydney's bio above.

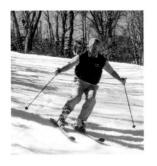

Jim Cottrell – has owed French Swiss Ski College for 35 years and has been a scratch golfer most of his adult life. Jim credits Jean Claude Kiley as his skiing mentor. He has published several books on skiing instruction and pre-season, "dry land ski school", ski training. As a golfer he is quick to say that putting is his weakness so his accurate (near perfect) iron game gets him closer to the hole. Thank you for your mentorship to me, and many others, over the years. Jim is a great man, a great role model for any young man, and has left an untold positive contribution to the skiing industry.

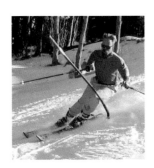

Jason Hegg – 2014 overall national second place Men's US amateur (NASTAR) in slalom ranking in the regular season. Jason finished 2nd place nationally in the 2015 male 35 - 39 amateur open category. Jason and his bother grew up in Duluth racing against Bodie Miller in the juniors. Thank you for the letting me take pictures of you in your golf attire on such a cold day. Moreover, taking one for the team by smashing his knee on a gate for the sake of the picture, the use of your camera and the camera tips. More importantly, you are a great friend and a great dad. Currently, Jason has a successful law practice in Jacksonville, North Carolina. A sharp lawyer, with an engineering degree, who can ski and is a great guy may be someone you want to call if needed. jhegglaw@gmail.com

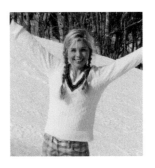

Madison Deering – she is a student, a gifted athlete and pursuing a career in professional modeling. She would be a stellar model or spokes model to represent any company, campaign, event or cause. Contact Sharon Dunn, SharonEDunn@att.net to book Madison. Thank you and your sister for the photo shoot day. I do not recall ever laughing so much on a ski day.

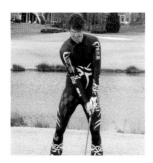

David Stewart – is one of the faster racers, better athletes, and nicest guys you ever meet. David works as successful commercial real estate developer and is dad of three boys. Thank you for your friendship and agreeing to put on your speed suit on the golf course in front of people you know for the photo shoot.

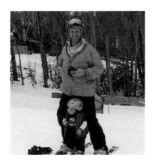

Chuck Vance and Troy Vance – By wining hundreds of races over the past thirty years, Chuck can easily be considered as one of the faster slalom racers to make a turn on the planet. I know our sport will be in good hands as he passes the passion for skiing onto Troy.

Other Thanks

Elizabeth Drake Boyt – Erete's Bloom Professional Editing Services - eddi47patt@gmail.com. This our second book together. In addition to her professionalism, effectiveness and prompt responsiveness, she is a joy to work with. She consistently exceeds my expectations. If you have need of a professional editor for a project or book, I would certainly recommend her services.

Tyler Hayes – Thanks for being my go-to graphic artist resource for over two years. Tyler created the Golfers and Skiers book cover and book formatting. He also created the cover on my first book – "Future Business Stars" © 2014 . Tyler is a brilliant and talented young man highly recommended. He is currently studying Graphic Design in the College of Design at North Carolina State University. If you need graphic arts professional services I recommend you contact Tyler at www.bytylerhayes.com. I am sure he will soon be with a large agency, cherry-picking the best and brightest talent once he graduates.

River Run County Club (Home of the Chiquita Classic) – for the use of their club for many of the golf pictures with David Ross, Cydney Clanton, the 19th hole picture, the golf gadgets, golf cart pictures, beer cart picture and the golf equipment picture .

Trump National County Club- Charlotte – for the use of their club for many golf pictures of Cydney Clanton.

French Swiss Ski College and Jim Cottrell and his staff - for all the help in help with the photo shoots and the complementary lift tickets for the model/skiers.

Lynn Wise – Professional copy proofing. I have worked with Lynn for over two years. Contact me if you want to use Lynn's services at mike@gamechangingbusinessskills.com.

Dr. John Priester – Doctor of Chiropractic - proof of concept review, technical review and encouragement. Also, for fixing me after my many racing skiing crashes for the past thirty years.

Martha Honeycutt – proof of concept review and editing.

Sarah Honeycutt – for the use of her speed suit in the photo shoots.

Perry Aliotti – former skiing instructor and avid golfer - editing, proof of concept, advice and encouragement.

Tom Rigsby – National Ski Patrol – Proof of Concept and editing.

Alpine Ski Center (Charlotte) – for the use of props for the pictures.

Sugar Mountain - for the use of their slopes for photo shoots.

Telluride Ski Resort - for the use of pictures. Thanks Patrick Rothe!

Snowshoe Ski Resort for the use of their slopes for photo shoots.

David Duncan with Liberty University for photo permissions.

Appalachian Ski Mountain - for the use of their slopes for several days of photo shoots. Thanks Jim Cottrell, the Moretz family and to the rest of the crew.

Ski Beech - for the use of their slopes for photo shoots. Thanks Ryan!

Mallard Head Golf Course - for allowing the photo of their club in this book.

Sherrie Durell - for the use of her photo.

Thanks to Crescent racers - The ski racing group picture includes Tricia Wall, Jessica Starr, Jason Hegg, Larry Sottile, David Stoner, Alex Jonker, Ryan Johnson, Ryan Langley, Jenny Pennington, Jake Grigorian, Cathy Mulgrew and Mike Dunn.

Steve Parris – for letting me take his picture at Mallard Head Golf Club.

Kirk Durell – Satirical Editor – words cannot express my thanks for your friendship and laughs over the years.

Steve Lambert – Marketing advice and encouragement.

Debra Funderburk – Book Marketing Consultant – Thanks so much for your valued advice and expertise. I look forward to working with you on many more projects.

Laurie Anne Alvine – Social Media Expert – Thanks for the help with my commercial Facebook, Instagram and Pinterest development.

Eryn Padgett – for letting me take her picture while making her rounds with her beer cart.

Sierra Deering – Help with a photo shoot.

John Gardner – Help with a photo shoot.

Candace Vance - for the use of her photo of Chuck and Troy Vance

Kirk Durell – for the hundreds of hours we spent together on all the least expensive golf courses in town while learning to play golf. Also, for Kirk and Sherrie for all the ski trips in the US and Europe.

Steve Lambert – for all the skiing trips to the Western resorts, Canada and our heli-skiing trip.

Chuck Vance - for all the racing weekends and time doing drills trying to teach me the details of a correct ski turn. It had to have been frustrating.

Patrick Rothe – for letting me follow you as we learned how to ski steep off-piste terrain. Also, for letting me visit you in Telluride during a few of my life's rough spots.

All my skiing friends over the years.

All my golfing friends over the years.

Most of all, thanks to my Dad, George Dunn, for teaching me the sport of golf.

Credits

Place where snowmaking was invented in Connecticut. "Making Snow". About.com. Retrieved 2006-12-16

Purchased pictures were acquired from www.istock.com and www.dreamstime.com

(USGA) is a registered trademark of the United States Golf Association

All Golf Statistics are courtesy of Golf info Guide by Thomas Golf. www.golf-info-guide.com   Thanks Sal!

Europe and worldwide ski data courtesy of www.J2Ski.com. Thanks David Pellatt.

US and worldwide skiing data courtesy of www.WhiteBookofSkiAreas.com Thanks David Schissler

Ski Area non text data - Wikipedia non text open data – 17 U.S.C 103B

(FIS) is a registered trademark of the International Ski Federation

Tyler Hayes – graphic art services for the book cover and book formatting.

"Best Snow on Earth" is a registered trademark of State of Utah

"In a balanced and athletic stance, you could ski down any mountain in the world… You just may not be able to stop" - Jim Cottrell

Fuxi refers to Fuxi Racing USA. www.fuxiracingusa.com

Charlotte Ski Team picture

Golfers & Skiers Order Form

Order here:

http://shop.golfersandskiers.com/Golfers-and-Skiers-Book_c2.htm

Order more books

Use the coupon code **FRIENDS** to buy:

One additional book for $5.00 off

Two books — $5.00 off the first book and 20% off the second

Three or more — 20% off the whole order

Christmas Shopping Easy Deal | Office Party Gift Easy Deal

8 books for $17.40 each - use coupon code "XMAS8" (includes shipping)

12 books for $16.99 each – use coupon code "XMAS12" (includes shipping)

Email me for larger quantities at mike@golfersandskiers.com and I'll gladly give you a great deal.

Gifts for your Golfers & Skiers

Shirts - Golfers and Skiers Tee shirts (cotton)

Classic looking style – white shirt with green lettering.

Sizes: Infant, child, small, medium, large, XL, XXL

Ball Caps

Classic very curved bill golf ball cap

Urban Style with straight bill ball cap

Contact me with questions or comments at mike@golfersandskiers.com

Printed in Great Britain
by Amazon